SPECI

MW01126645

STOP SEX ADDICTION
Real Hope, True Freedom for Sex Addicts and Partners

"The most comprehensive text since *Out of the Shadows*.
A must-read for every sex addict, their partner, and their family.
Each page instills hope for those struggling with sexual addiction,
while not minimizing the pain involved in the process.
It will help newcomers and old-timers alike."

David L. Delmonico, PhD
Author of *In the Shadows of the Net*
and *Cybersex Unhooked*

. . .

"Writing from a wealth of experience, Milton Magness has
written a superb book to both partners in a relationship impacted
by sex addiction. He clearly grasps the depth and breadth of the
problem, doesn't minimize the profound impact, and at the same
time offers the reader hope. The addicted person and his or her partner
will both feel understood, supported, and validated. Without detracting
from the reader who is personally affected, Magness also offers clinical
direction to the treatment professional. You feel him speaking to the
readers and know he is championing them in their journey."

Claudia Black, PhD, Addiction Specialist
Author of *Intimate Treason* and *Deceived*

. . .

"I've worked with many women who, along with their partner, have done a weekend intensive with Dr. Magness, and I consistently see these marriages having higher success rates than the ones that don't utilize his services. I'm delighted that now, between the covers of this book, many more couples and individuals will be able to take advantage of his wisdom, experience, and guidance as they grapple with sexual addiction in their lives and marriages. This is a must-read for anyone who falls into that painful category, and for everyone who seeks to help others dealing with this issue in their lives. I often tell people this is the only book they really need to read if they want to know about sexual addiction. It is the best 'bible' on the subject."

Marsha Means, MA
Author of *Living with Your Husband's Secret Wars*
and Co-author of *Your Sexually Addicted Spouse*

. . .

"This book is a very helpful tool for therapists and for people who are either having challenges with sexual addiction or have partners or friends who have that pain in their lives caused by relationships with sexual addicts. It is a very balanced, hopeful, clinically sound resource and gives very specific guidance as a map for holistic spiritual growth. We recommend this book to our patients at PCS. Dr. Milton Magness invites us into his therapy world with this book."

Ralph H. Earle, PhD
Author of *The Pornography Trap*,
Lonely All the Time, and Co-author of *Sex Addiction*

. . .

"In his new book, Dr. Magness expertly navigates the complexities of sexual addiction, while simultaneously making the reality of this intimacy disorder understandable for individuals who suffer, partners who love them, and those in the clinical community who are trying to help. This is currently the most thorough resource available for those of us concerned about the reality of sexual addiction. A must-read!"

Kelly McDaniel, MA
Author of *Ready to Heal*

STOP SEX ADDICTION

STOP SEX ADDICTION

REAL HOPE, TRUE FREEDOM FOR SEX ADDICTS AND PARTNERS

MILTON S. MAGNESS

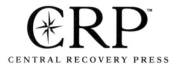

CENTRAL RECOVERY PRESS

Central Recovery Press (CRP) is committed to publishing exceptional materials addressing addiction treatment, recovery, and behavioral healthcare topics, including original and quality books, audio/visual communications, and web-based new media. Through a diverse selection of titles, we seek to contribute a broad range of unique resources for professionals, recovering individuals and their families, and the general public.

For more information, visit **www.centralrecoverypress.com.**

Central Recovery Press, Las Vegas, NV 89129

Publisher: Central Recovery Press
             3321 N. Buffalo Drive
             Las Vegas, NV 89129

18 17 16 15 14 13   1 2 3 4 5

ISBN-13: 978-1-937612-23-8 (paper)
ISBN-13: 978-1-937612-24-5 (e-book)

Author photo by Ocean Images. Used with permission.

Publisher's Note: This book contains general information about sex addiction and its effects on relationships. Central Recovery Press makes no representations or warranties in relation to the information herein; it is not an alternative to medical advice from your doctor or other professional healthcare provider.

Our books represent the experiences and opinions of their authors only. Every effort has been made to ensure that events, institutions, and statistics presented in our books as facts are accurate and up-to-date. To protect their privacy, some of the names of people and institutions have been changed.

Author's Note: The approach used in this book reflects the treatment model that is used at Hope & Freedom Counseling Services as well by Certified Hope & Freedom Practitioners (CHFP) who have been trained in the Hope & Freedom treatment model.

Cover design and interior design and layout by Sara Streifel, Think Creative Design

To my wife, Kathie,

who is the inspiration behind

Hope & Freedom

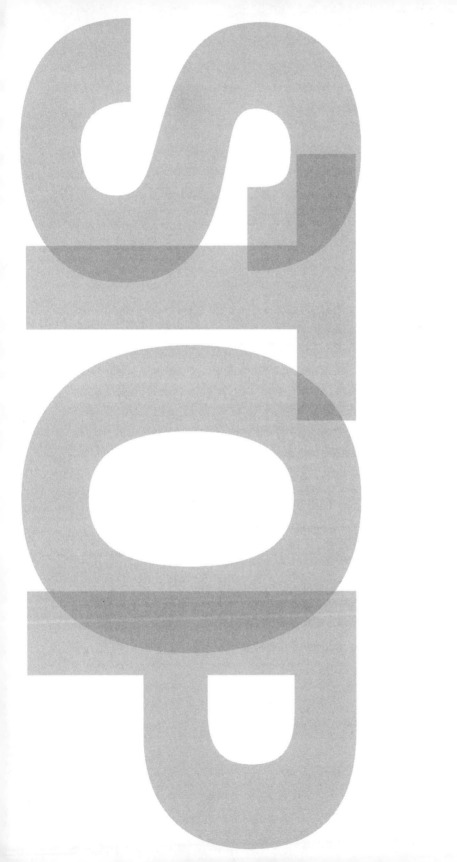

TABLE OF CONTENTS

PREFACE

The crisis that caused you to open this book is a true gift. In the middle of your present pain you may not see it as a gift. But as you take this recovery journey, you can get your life back.

This journey is an odyssey. You need to recognize at the outset that this is not a quick trip. It is an expedition that lasts a lifetime.

This book is about hope and, ultimately, freedom. Problematic sexual behavior, or sex addiction, is often difficult to face. Sex addiction results in countless negative consequences and hurts many people. Marriages and careers are destroyed by sex addiction.

There is hope because sex addiction is treatable. Through hard work and a rigorous recovery program, it is possible for sex addicts to stop all their destructive behaviors forever, and for marriages and other relationships to be restored. The recovery road is long and difficult but also very rewarding.

Whether you are a sex addict or the person you love is a sex addict, you can find help within this book. I engage in psychotherapy with sex addicts and their spouses and loved ones because I see lives and relationships transformed daily. Some consider recovery to be the result of hard work alone. But I see it as a miracle, and I get to see miracles happen every day. Individuals who were once powerless to resist destructive behaviors overcome them. Marriages and other relationships on the brink of divorce or dissolution can be restored, with trust reestablished.

If you are a sex addict, or have a crisis caused by your partner's problematic sexual behavior, this book is for you. Numerous sex addicts who thought they could not stop acting out have made a permanent break with their problematic sexual behavior. My goal is to bring you a message of hope and a way to achieve freedom, honesty, and renewed trust in yourself and with the person you love.

Recovery is not something one *has* to do, but something one gets to do! If you can make that mental shift as you read this book and see recovery as a gift instead of a penalty for bad behavior, you will be in a position to make extraordinary gains in your personal life. Recovery is a gift that comes from the hard work needed to replace dysfunctional thoughts and behaviors. It builds a foundation upon which trust can be restored, leads to freedom from all problematic sexual behavior, and restores badly damaged relationships.

This book is addressed to sex addicts and partners. While a larger percentage of sex addicts are men, women also fall victim to this form of addiction. Access to the Internet in particular has made it easy for women to engage in acting-out behaviors. This book pertains to both genders.

In late October of 2011, Hope & Freedom Counseling Services sent out a survey to partners of sex addicts. The original intent of the survey was to gather information for a video series (www.imustheal.com) that was developed as an adjunct to this book. One hundred and three partners or former partners of sex addicts chose to participate, and their responses were compiled in January of 2012. Those who completed the survey shared an incredible amount of information. They spent, on average, thirty-three and a half minutes each completing the surveys. The wisdom they shared is contained in this book; specific survey results are discussed in Chapters 14, 17, and 19.

By following the steps described in this book, addicts and their partners can find the path to freedom from sex addiction. A Chinese adage states that the hardest part of any journey is the first step. You have already begun that journey by picking up this book. Continue reading, follow the guidance contained herein, and I believe your life will change.

ACKNOWLEDGMENTS

There are several people who have had a significant impact on my life since I founded Hope & Freedom Counseling Services and also while writing this book.

Dr. Ralph Earle and Dr. Marcus Earle from Psychological Counseling Services in Scottsdale, Arizona, have always been most gracious with their encouragement. I owe much of what Hope & Freedom has become to ideas I have borrowed from you.

I would especially like to thank Marsha Means with A Circle of Joy for the very significant work that she does with the many wounded spouses of sex addicts. Your gifted work with traumatized spouses has made the work I do with couples much more effective. It is always a pleasure to collaborate with you in working with couples who are hurting.

I also wish to thank the many gifted colleagues who have made an impact on my life, including Adam Mason, Greg Curnutte, Huston McComb, Enie Bourland, Doug Sorensen, Tim Mavergeorge, Cara Weed, Tim Lee, Dr. Alexis Llewellyn, Jerry Goodman, Enod Gray, Dr. Barbara Levinson, Joni Ogle, Sylvia Jason, and Karen Thomas. In addition, I would like to thank Dr. Vicki Wyatt, who took a chance on our new training program and became the first therapist certified to incorporate the Hope & Freedom treatment model into her practice.

I especially want to thank Sara Streifel of Think Creative Design for book and cover design, and the great team at Central Recovery Press including Dan Mager for his editing skill, and Patrick Hughes for his marketing expertise; and a special thanks to Nicole Thomas and Nancy Schenck for their patience and persistence in helping me make the transition to a new publisher. I hope we have the opportunity to work on additional projects together.

Finally, I appreciate the impassioned responses of the partners of sex addicts who responded to our survey. Your experiences, your wisdom, and your hope added significantly to this book. And of course, I wish to thank the many men and women who have come to Hope & Freedom's Three-Day Intensive program. It has been a privilege to be a part of your recovery journey. I pray that you may continue to live in hope and freedom and that you will find full restoration to your relationship. Recovery can truly be a wonderful adventure!

CHAPTER 1

SEX ADDICTION IN AMERICA

Sex addiction is a growing menace that threatens all strata of our society. Former presidents, governors, senators, leading actors, senior executives, and other high-profile persons have been disgraced when they admitted they were involved in some secret sexual behavior. Ministers, priests, doctors, lawyers, teachers, and community leaders have seen their careers cut short when they were caught in compromising sexual behaviors. Millions of marriages and relationships have been ruined or ended. Numerous reputations have been sacrificed on the altar of problematic sexual behavior. Because some sexual behavior is illegal, many have been sent to prison. Some have taken their own lives rather than face the embarrassment of prosecution. Although not as well-known as other forms of addiction such as alcohol, drugs, and gambling, sex addiction is responsible for the waste of billions of dollars annually.

Worldwide pornography revenues exceed $97 billion per year.[1] This number would certainly be higher were it not for the fact that there is so much free pornography available on the Internet. In the United States the revenue generated annually by pornography exceeds the combined revenue of ABC, CBS, and NBC. A conservative estimate is that pornography generates at least $10 billion in the United States each year. That is about the same amount that Americans pay for sporting events and concerts combined. There are other costs that figure into the cost of sex addiction. There have been multiple lawsuits against the Catholic Church for sexual abuse of minors. The church has spent more than $2.6 billion in settlement costs and related expenses since 1950.[2] There are more than twelve million people exploited by trafficking in the sex trade.[3] Annual costs of medical treatment for sexually transmitted diseases in the United States exceeds $15.3 billion.[4]

Rafael's Story
Rafael was often told that he was attractive. When single, he was always able to get dates and had his pick of cute women. He had been in a committed relationship for two years. Fourteen months ago, he drove past a lovely young woman and offered her a ride. She asked him if he would like a date. He found out her idea of a "date" was that she was willing to be sexual with him as long as he was willing to give her shopping money.

That was his first experience with a prostitute. He started picking up prostitutes in those parts of the city frequented by them. He fancied himself a negotiator and would sometimes spend the entire day propositioning various prostitutes for sex acts and trying to see how cheaply he could make the deal. His behavior sometimes put him at risk because these areas of his city were also drug-infested and had a high incidence of violent crime. I have spent years treating sex addicts like Rafael, and encounter individuals from every walk of life, educational background, and social standing. While every individual is unique, the common denominator is overwhelming despair as a result of being unable to control one's addiction or the sadness of seeing one's spouse in the throes of addiction. I have hundreds of heart-wrenching emails from people reaching out for help. The following are quotes from a sample of these pleas:

From a woman: *"Sexual addiction is ruining my life and I need your help. Sometimes I'll go out and pick up a guy, have sex with him, then go home to have sex with my husband . . . all in the same evening. I have been known to fly across the country to have sex with people I haven't even met face-to-face. I have had sex with my therapist, my doctor, my dentist, and even my brother. The list is endless. Please help me."*

From a man: *"I am just about 100 percent certain that I am a sex addict and feel I need immediate help, as I feel it is ruining my life. It is very hard for me to concentrate on anything other than sex."*

A wife's heartfelt concern: *"Please tell me where I can get help for my husband. He has been a sex addict for the past ten years. We have three beautiful children. I recently discovered a secret phone with the phone numbers of many different women, and there were condoms hidden with it. Please help me."*

A worried father: *"I have a son who began watching hard-core pornography clips on the Internet about two years ago. Now he is doing it again. I am concerned that he will grow up as an addict."*

No profession is spared from sex addiction: *"I am an ordained minister and married with two children. For years now I have struggled with same-gender attraction. I am attracted to my wife physically and sexually, and yet at the same time I find myself fighting attraction to men. Although I struggle with addiction to gay pornography and sex toys, I feel sick whenever I give in to temptation, but I cannot stop."*

Sex addiction manifests itself in an extensive variety of behaviors or acting out. One man wrote: *"I am fighting this sexual addiction of dressing* up and wanting to escalate my fantasies. My wife and children have no clue as to what has been consuming me."

The addict's pain is always palpable: "I'm a longtime sex and pornography addict. I've been to counselors piled on top of more counselors. This very day, I've hit bad websites and acted out. I've been married to an angel for eleven years. It hurts. I'd be lying if I said it didn't."

Sometimes help comes too late: "My wife is planning to leave me because I can't stop looking at porn. I spend a lot of time on the computer looking at porn. It is constantly in the way of my relationship with my wife, and I'm going to lose her."

The son of a doctor wrote: "My father was caught with explicit pictures of his patients and is facing criminal charges. He and my mom need immediate counseling to help in this crisis."

One letter states the problem as a desire to be free from addiction, yet denies the addiction: "I have lost my wife and home, can't keep a job. I deny I have a problem, yet my life is so out of control and stays that way. Why is that and what should I do?"

Palmer's Story

Travel was a way of life for Palmer. While he was out of town, his acting out was viewing Internet pornography and pay-per-view adult movies he could access from hotels. He had been sexually sober on and off for three years. Palmer attended meetings and even had a sponsor, but felt he was not like other sex addicts because his acting out had consisted primarily of Internet pornography and compulsive masturbation.

He had just gone to his favorite acting-out website when someone knocked on the door. He opened the door just a crack, and a hotel maid asked if she could put fresh towels in the bathroom. When she saw what he had been doing, she propositioned him and offered to have sex with him in his room. He was initially shocked and *thought about telling management. Later on that same trip, the idea excited him, and he had sex with the same maid and paid her for her services.*

That was the beginning of a pattern for Palmer of checking into hotels and making leading comments to hotel maids to see if he could find one willing to be sexual with him. Sometimes he was successful, but most of the time he was not. He felt this was a low-risk behavior because even if he was turned down, he doubted that he would be reported. He believed that people in low-wage jobs would be reluctant to report something that could end up costing them their job.

As his courage grew, even when not traveling he used the same technique of preying on unsuspecting women he thought would be vulnerable because of their low wages. He would especially target women working in parking booths at airports and cashiers at grocery stores. Sometimes he scored. Sometimes he struck out. He was always on the hunt. The pursuit consumed him.

Such cases are not isolated examples of sexual addiction. The Society for the Advancement of Sexual Health (SASH), the international organization of sex addiction therapists, has concluded that between 3 and 5 percent of the people in the United States are sexually addicted.[5] Since this number is based on those who have sought treatment for their problem sexual behaviors, many sex addiction therapists believe the true number is significantly higher. What lies below the surface is a terrifying image of unchecked sexual impulses impacting the morals of society.

What Is Sex Addiction?

Depending on a person's perspective, he or she may have many different understandings of sex addiction. The uninitiated person may think of sex addiction as being synonymous with sex offending or predation. But interestingly enough, most sex addicts are not sex offenders or predators, and most sex offenders and predators do not meet the clinical criteria for sex addiction.

Uninformed people have been known to say, "If I ever have a form of addiction, I want it to be sex addiction." But a person who suffers from sex addiction knows that this is not a disorder to be desired or made light of. A person suffering from sex addiction has most likely tried numerous times to address his or her destructive behaviors.

In defining sex addiction, it might be helpful to consider what it is not. Someone is not a sex addict just because he or she likes to have sex or wants to have sex often. One woman told me that her thirty-five-year-old husband must be a sex addict "because he wants to have sex every day." Actually, the frequency with which a person has sex has little to do with the diagnosis of sex addiction. It is possible for a person to have sex very frequently and not be a sex addict. And it is possible for a person to have sex very infrequently but still be a sex addict.

Sex addiction is also not synonymous with infidelity. Just because a person has been unfaithful does not automatically mean he or she is a sex addict. It is even possible for a married person to have been unfaithful multiple times and still not be a sex addict.

In a similar fashion, sex addiction is not defined by any particular behavior. Some might want to say someone is a sex addict because that person visited a prostitute, went to a strip club, or viewed hardcore pornography on the Internet. But the presence of any or even all of these things is not enough to diagnose someone as a sex addict.

Sex addiction is described by many different names. In addition to sex addiction, it is called problematic sexual behavior, compulsive sexual behavior, sexual compulsivity, hypersexual behavioral disorder, or hypersexual disorder.

Sex addiction can be defined a number of ways. A basic definition is that sex addiction is an intimacy disorder characterized by compulsive thoughts or actions. Other definitions include things like distress over a pattern of repeated sexual behaviors, or excessive sex drive.

My definition is this: Sex addiction is a progressive intimacy disorder whereby a person engages in a pattern of sexual thoughts or behaviors that are destructive and that the person feels he or she is unable to stop.

Some sex addicts signal by their conversation, by their facial expressions, by their eye contact, or by the use of touch that they are available and would welcome an advance. Then they claim to be innocent, saying that they never initiated any of the affairs that resulted: "Women just always flirt with me." If this describes you, it is time for you to take in the welcome mat. And it is time to get honest about your behavior!

The fact that this is a recognizable disorder is also a starting place for hope. This disorder is treatable. And if you suffer from sex addiction, I want you to know that you do not have to stay as you are. The person who embarks on the road to recovery from sex addiction finds that this road can lead to the chance to begin again! You have started down that road. Finding this road has been painful. Maybe all you can see is pain and misery like that which you have already encountered.

Keep moving forward. If you do, in only a few weeks you will begin to see some of the wonder that is waiting for you.

CHAPTER 2

HIERARCHY OF SEX ADDICTION

Benjamin's Story

Benjamin and his wife had been married three years when he told her that he had always had a fantasy of watching her have sex with another man. She had a negative visceral reaction to his fantasy and told him that would never happen. From time to time he reminded her of his fantasy and then asked if she would be willing to at least participate in the fantasy by saying shocking things to him while they were having sex. Benjamin continued to manipulate her and ask her to tell him how much she wanted to fulfill his fantasy.

While on a romantic weekend getaway, Benjamin convinced her to participate in a couples erotic massage in their hotel room.

Prior to the massage they were drinking heavily. She did not know that Benjamin had already told the man who was coming to do the massage that he wanted him to have sex with his wife. In her drunken state, and with the pressure from Benjamin and the other man, she relented and had intercourse with this man while her husband watched. The next day she was devastated by what she had done. She knew her husband had taken advantage of her. She was angry that her husband thought so little of her that he violated clear boundaries that she had set.

Several weeks later Benjamin was shocked when he was served with divorce papers. He had no idea that his wife would react so badly to what he thought was a natural extension of his fantasy. Benjamin has started seeing a therapist and is attending twelve-step meetings in an effort to save his marriage, which may not be salvageable. The fact that he is now in recovery is a step in the right direction. But for Benjamin to be truly successful in recovery in the long term, he must make a mental shift and participate actively in the recovery process for himself, regardless of what happens in his relationship.

Although sex addiction has yet to be included in the *Diagnostic and Statistical Manual of Mental Disorders (DSM-IV-TR)*,[6] the reference manual for all psychiatric and behavioral health conditions, there is widespread acknowledgment among professionals of the ways its symptoms are comparable to other forms of addiction. As with mind- and mood-altering substances and drug addiction, for those struggling with sex addiction sex offers a quick mood change, while the user loses control over his or her increasingly compulsive behavior. Like those with other forms of addiction, sex addicts construct their lives around the need for their drug: sex.

With those addicted to alcohol and other drugs, there are undeniable signs of abuse and immediate penalties, such as arrest for DUI or public intoxication. Addiction involving alcohol is more socially overt than other forms of addiction in terms of the availability of alcohol in public establishments such as bars and stores. Illicit drugs, including abused prescription medications, are more clandestine in terms of purchase and use. They quickly betray the addict who uses them. Moreover, in the case of substances, the hangover or come-down aftereffects have significant physical as well as psychological impacts.

Sex addiction is more subtle in the ways it can be experienced and maintained. It can take many forms—compulsive masturbation, viewing pornography, or being sexual with other people. Others may express their sex addiction by becoming involved in illegal activities, such as solicitation of prostitution, exhibitionism, or voyeurism. The common denominator is that all sex addicts feel driven to participate in their sexual behavior regardless of the risk and potential consequences.

The Society for the Advancement of Sexual Health defines several recurring components of sex addiction: "Compulsivity, a loss of the ability to choose freely whether to stop or to continue; continuation of the behavior despite adverse consequences, such as loss of health, marriage, or freedom; and obsession with the activity."[7]

Unlike addiction to substances that is limited to drugs including alcohol, sex addiction is not limited in the way it may be acted out, and can even occur entirely within the imagination, such as thinking about women in swimsuits at a beach, or fantasizing a sexual scene while driving. As undetectable as are some forms of imagined sexual addiction, the most common visible forms are recognizable:

• Sexual promiscuity.

• Viewing pornography.

• Frequenting sex-oriented businesses like massage parlors, "gentlemen's clubs" (talk about a euphemism!), modeling studios, video arcades, and "sex toy" stores.

• Prostitution.

• Exhibitionism.

• Voyeurism.

The term "sex addiction" is often misunderstood. For some, realizing there is a name for out-of-control sexual behavior is a relief. It helps explain why a person will continue the behavior, knowing the great risks to his or her relationship, health, job/career, or freedom. For others, the term feels like a label charged with negative implications and without hope.

Aaron's Story

Aaron would not consider living an openly gay lifestyle because it conflicts with his conservative religious beliefs. He always suspected that he was gay but has never been able to reconcile his beliefs with his actions. He has been successful hiding his sexual behavior from everyone he knows.

As far as his friends know, he is a single man who occasionally has dates with women but prefers to remain single. What his friends do not know is that Aaron has engaged in secret sexual rendezvous with men for many years. Most consist of anonymous encounters with strangers. He struggles with guilt over his sexual behavior but feels powerless to stop.

Gay or straight, male or female, sex addiction is an equal-opportunity form of addiction. Although sex addiction is not considered a diagnosable disorder by some mental health professionals, for the person who suffers from it or is in a relationship with someone who suffers from it, there is no question that it is a legitimate affliction. If you prefer the term *hypersexuality* or *sexual compulsivity disorder*, then mentally insert your term each time you see the term *sex addiction* in this book. From my clinical experience, I believe sex addiction is a valid disorder affecting many people.

William's Story

William was in his second year of medical school when he found a sex chat room while looking for something to break the monotony of studying. To his surprise, he found people who were very open about their sexual desires and behaviors. To say that he was captivated by what he saw would be an understatement. After a few hours of what William thought was a harmless diversion, he went back to his studies.

The next night he was back in the chat room and ended up spending much more time than he intended. Short on sleep, he went to class the next day but fell further behind. In the evening he sought comfort in various chat rooms. Somehow he managed to successfully complete the school year, but he realized that his cybersex behaviors were becoming hard to control.

William tried to stop but found himself back in the chat rooms after a hiatus of only a few days. The third year of med school was the most challenging yet. Rather than being able to meet the challenge, he retreated into the comfortable and predictable cybersex behavior that made him forget the pressure of school for hours at a time. Each day he would look forward to the end of his classes when he was able to escape into his fantasy world. To his dismay, William fell hopelessly behind on his assignments. Even after being shown significant leniency by his professors, he knew he would not be able to catch up. Finally the dean asked him to withdraw from school and save himself the embarrassment of flunking out. How could this happen? His grades in high school and college were always at the top of the class. He had one of the highest scores ever on his entrance exam. The only thing that explains William's dramatic fall was that he was firmly in the clutches of sex addiction.

About one in twenty people meet the clinical criteria for addiction. It could be as high as one in ten. Using the more conservative figure means that there are as many sex addicts in the United States as there are people with bipolar disorder, obsessive-compulsive disorder, panic disorder, and schizophrenia combined. Put another way, there are as many sex addicts in the United States as people living in New York, Chicago, Los Angeles, Houston, and Boston combined!

A casual review of today's media confirms the extent of disruptive and destructive problematic sexual behavior going on daily. Much of what passes for entertainment on TV, in movies, and in comedy clubs is sexual in nature. It is harmful when sex addiction is portrayed as humorous. One wonders what would happen if innuendo and more explicit content related to sex and problematic sexual behavior were removed from our avenues of entertainment.

Brian's Story

Brian has a secret he has never told anyone. He has a fetish with women's panties. It began when he was thirteen. He found a pair of his older sister's panties in the bathroom. He was fascinated by the material and the construction of the underwear that was so different from his briefs. He kept the panties in his room and would sometimes wear them while he masturbated. As he grew older he would look for opportunities to steal underwear from his sister's friends. When he would have sleepovers at his friends' houses, he would go through their sisters' and mothers' bureaus as well as their dirty clothes hampers, adding to his panty collection.

Over the years he has spent a lot of time cruising laundry rooms in apartment complexes, looking for unattended dryers that may contain underwear. He has frequently bought lingerie that he asks his sexual partners to wear. While they usually accommodate his requests, some are irritated because he seems more interested in their underwear than their bodies. A couple of his partners have caught him trying to steal their underwear, and once he was chased out of the laundry room at an apartment complex by a guard who had been alerted to his odd behavior. In spite of the potential consequences, he does not believe it is possible for him to stop stealing panties. Although he purchases some of his underwear, he gets a higher sexual arousal from stealing them.

A variety of problematic sexual behaviors may be present in people addicted to sex. There are several hundred identified problematic sexual behaviors. This list names just a few:

- Compulsive masturbation, sometimes to the point of injury.

- Renting or purchasing pornographic photographs, movies, games, and/or magazines.

- Engaging in cybersex behaviors such as exchanging sexual emails, frequenting chat rooms, and using webcams to engage in mutual masturbation or exhibitionism.

- Engaging in phone sex.

- Frequenting sex-oriented businesses (such as strip clubs, sexual massage parlors, modeling studios, bathhouses, and adult bookstores or arcades).

- Having sex with prostitutes.

- Engaging in sex in exchange for payment.

- Carrying on multiple relationships at once.

- Having anonymous sex.

- Engaging in sadomasochistic or "pain exchange" sex.

- Using drugs, including alcohol, to heighten sexual euphoria.

- Exhibitionism.

- Voyeurism.

- Professional-boundary violations (as with physicians, attorneys, therapists, and clergy).

- Indecent phone calls.

- Touching people in a sexual manner without their permission, which is known as *frotteurism*.

While a higher percentage of men traditionally act out these forms of behavior, more women are entering into arenas of sex addiction. The presence of one or several sexual behaviors is not proof that a person is a sex addict. Certainly, sexual behaviors outside of a marriage or committed relationship predicated on monogamy damages the relationship. A number of factors must be considered before an individual can be diagnosed as a sex addict.

Symptoms of Sex Addiction

Problematic sexual behaviors provide a way for some people to medicate their feelings and cope with stress. As with drugs that are used for the same purposes, sex is effective in temporarily avoiding pain. The continuing use of sex as self-medication for stress and loneliness requires more frequent sexual acting out and/or riskier behavior to achieve the same relief as before.

Those addicted to sex find themselves unable to control, limit, or moderate their behavior. They may use inordinate amounts of time to pursue their addiction. Trying to control their behavior, they make promises to themselves and to those they love, and even make vows to God, that they will stop. But they are unable to do so.

Among some spiritual people, sex addiction may be an effort to fill a void in their life that only God can fill. Even religious persons having a personal relationship with God may use sex to try to give their lives more meaning. With each sexual encounter they find temporary relief from loneliness or low self-esteem. But they find that their "fix" lasts for shorter durations each time, necessitating an escalation in their addictive behavior in order to feel relief again. A typical course of sex addiction includes an escalation of behaviors and the development of an increased tolerance, requiring more sex or more extreme sexual behavior in order for the sex addict to be satisfied.

Sex addicts may isolate themselves from others, sometimes to the point of having little or no contact with people. They may find their primary sexual outlet with pornography or cybersex activities and not want to risk rejection that could come from moving from the omnipotent power in a virtual landscape to a world of living human beings with their own emotional needs.

Sex addicts typically feel that their lives are out of control. They may experience a loss of time, where they find many hours passing during their acting out but feel that only a few minutes have passed. Sex addicts habitually use dishonesty to provide cover for their activities. Persons who are otherwise uncompromisingly honest may engage in blatant fabrications and contrived excuses to cover up their sexual behavior, as well as the time and money expended in their sexual pursuits.

As with addiction to substances, some sex addicts suffer withdrawal symptoms if they are unable to act out. Withdrawal symptoms may include restlessness, irritability, insomnia, and such a preoccupation with sex that they are unable to function at their job or with their family.

The presence of several of these symptoms may be an indication that a person is a sex addict. For a more accurate diagnosis, one should seek a psychotherapist skilled in diagnosing and treating sex addiction, or contact any of the organizations dealing with sex addiction found in the reference section at the end of this book.

In cases where a companion has admitted to being a sex addict but has not explained the reason for the behavior, the partner is left to wonder what sexual acting out is taking place when they are not together. He or she may wonder what else his or her partner is doing. The descriptions of sex addiction contained herein are intended to enlighten, not to offend. They are provided to help you understand the types of sexual behaviors common to this form of addiction. Please note that every sex addict is not involved in every behavior discussed here. Many examples are given to inform you of the breadth of this disorder and to help you discern if you or someone you love may be suffering from it.

Robbie's Story

Robbie manages a successful hedge fund. He is always under pressure to perform and produce results for his clients. For a change of pace during the day, he will occasionally turn to the Internet and spend a few minutes acting out. These forays into fantasy have lately occupied more of his time. He first discovered virtual 3-D websites a couple of years ago. Robbie loved to go to those sites, adopt a fictional identity, and follow his made-up character through the normal routines of life.

Gradually, he moved from the ordinary routines of life to developing elaborate fictional characters, or avatars, to allow him to live out his sexual fantasies online. At first he would pretend to be the man he thought women would like. He then had fantasy sex with them. Robbie soon found more excitement by becoming the object of his affection. Since his ideal sex partners are twenty-four-year-old petite blondes, he decided to take on the role of various young women and then vicariously find sexual fulfillment through them.

To make his avatar more convincing, Robbie would spend many hours each week creating the perfect profile. He would scour various pornography sites and social networking sites for photos of young women who fit his ideal. To make the most credible profiles, he felt he needed not only nude photos of young women but also photos of them going through daily life, visiting with family and friends. There were weeks when Robbie spent more hours developing elaborate profiles than working at his job. After spending a few hours acting out with each avatar he created, he would start developing a new character that would be his obsession for the following week.

As a result of acting out, Robbie lost key clients, and his hedge fund is performing well below the market. With the increased pressure to perform at a higher level, he turned more frequently to his virtual world, which resulted in even poorer performance. Robbie knows he has to stop his acting out completely or he will destroy his business. However, he is unable to stop his self-destructive behavior.

The Dangers of Anonymity

Advances in technology have made it easy for sex addicts to act out with less chance of discovery. Virtual websites such as Second Life and EverQuest allow members to engage virtually in many forms of sexual behavior with others while remaining anonymous, even to the extent of changing sexes. Acting out is achieved through an avatar. The same thing occurs with numerous video game consoles where players engage in virtual sex with those they compete against online. This is an increasingly dangerous behavior that has become addictive, especially to teens and young adults.

The virtual world creates temptation for sex addicts and pain for their real-world partners. At the time of this writing there are about 4.2 million pornographic websites. It is estimated that there are about 420 million pornographic pages on the Internet. Twenty-five percent of all search engine requests are for pornographic material. And 42.7 percent of all Internet users admit to viewing pornography.[8]

On the Internet anything goes, and sex addicts can act out with ease. As long as they can conceal their activities from spouses, employers, or peers, addiction is fostered. When they are caught, lives and relationships are often destroyed.

Individuals may be engaging in sexually addictive behavior online, thinking that because they are not in direct contact with others, there is no danger to them or their partner. They are mistaken. Sex addiction leads to emotional distance from loved ones and lying and deceit to conceal the addiction. Shame and guilt are constant companions. The impact goes beyond acting out in private. The cost to employers from workers using company time to visit pornographic websites is substantial. But the greatest damage addicts do is to themselves by hiding their addiction until it overtakes their life.

No technological advancement has done more to facilitate sex addiction than the Internet. It provides multiple opportunities to act out sexually and is a powerful accelerant to sexual addiction. The late Dr. Al Cooper, a researcher at Stanford University, stated that there are people who are sex addicts today who would never have been addicted were it not for the Internet. Access to the Internet makes things available at home that were previously only available in seedy adult entertainment establishments.

Have you ever wondered if religious faith builds immunity to the negative impact of pornography? Lifeway Research conducted a survey of 1,000 Protestant ministers in October of 2010.[9] Forty-nine percent of those surveyed strongly agreed that pornography has adversely affected the lives of their church members. Another 32 percent said they somewhat agree with that statement.

Dr. Cooper has explained the addictive power of the Internet in what he called the Triple A Engine. The Internet is Available: anyone can access it from home or a computer anywhere in the world. It is Affordable: for little cost or in many cases free, and pornographic images can be viewed, catalogued, and saved for additional viewing later. Many sex addicts want to make clear that they "never paid for any Internet pornography" as if they are less of an addict because they did not spend money for their pornography. Finally, it is Anonymous: rather than having to enter an adult establishment and risk being recognized by one's neighbors, it is possible to peruse the Internet in relative anonymity.[10]

The primary activity of sex addicts on the Internet is viewing pornography. These images may be photos, movies, or cartoons. Few are as relatively tame as the airbrushed photos associated with *Playboy* or *Playgirl* magazines. Rather, the pornography of the Internet is more graphic, more hard-core, and provides a neurochemical release of such magnitude that it is often instantly addictive to the viewer. Things that many people never dreamed of are depicted with such detail that nothing is left to the imagination.

Internet pornography ranges from explicit photos or movies of people having sex to acts involving heterosexual and homosexual sex, sex in single and group situations, sex involving foreign objects, sex with body fluids and waste, sex with animals, sex with children, and any conceivable fetish. That is not to say that everyone looking at Internet pornography is looking at all of these things, but rather that anything that a person can possibly imagine can be found on the Internet.

There are millions of free pornographic images on the Internet; however, pornographers are in the business to make money. They sell subscriptions to their sites where subscribers are allowed to return to the site at will without paying additional fees. Some sites take credit card or PayPal charges that often show up on one's bill as a seemingly innocuous charge. Frequently companies are identified by initials or are disguised to resemble legitimate businesses. Charges range from $10 to $50 or more. The charges may be a onetime event or be set up to automatically charge the card as a monthly subscription. While subscription fees are common, paid advertising accounts for a large percentage of revenues as well. Internet advances that include streaming video and easy-pay systems have been pioneered by the pornography industry. This industry is so lucrative and growing so rapidly that any figures describing its size are out of date before they are printed.

Another addictive sexual behavior involving the Internet is sexually explicit chat. Numerous services provide "adult chat rooms" that are specific to a person's individual proclivity. The categories include things like "Married but Looking," "Barely Legal," "Steamy Seniors," or other provocative and often pornographic titles.

Acting out with smartphones is increasing dramatically. An ever-growing number of apps are available for locating acting-out partners. Some of these apps are specifically for married people who want to cheat on their spouses. Others are for people who want to act out with other people of the same gender. There are apps that utilize the GPS function of smartphones to locate potential acting-out partners who may be nearby.

Jackie's Story

Jackie has been married to the same man for almost twenty years. A few years ago she believed that she might have missed something in life because she did not have any of the excitement that she craved. She started entertaining herself by going to chat rooms that were advertised for people who were "married but looking." Jackie had no intention of ever doing more than talking to the men she met online.

In chat rooms she could portray herself as the person that she secretly wanted to be. And to her surprise, there were always men who wanted to talk with her, and most suggested that they meet in person. Not wanting to be physically unfaithful to her husband, she successfully deflected all of the requests for face-to-face meetings. At least she deflected them until she decided to meet someone who insisted that she reminded him of his old high school girlfriend.

Before long, she was regularly engaging in secret meetings with men whom she would first contact in the chat rooms and then meet at secret locations. What started as a seemingly harmless diversion ended up becoming a full-blown sexual addiction, and ultimately led to divorce.

Chat rooms provide an open forum for people to meet and post electronic messages that can be seen by others in the "room." Each person in the room uses an identifier known as a "handle" rather than his or her real name. In sex chat rooms it is common to see handles like "Hot to Trot in Tulsa" or "Sexy and Ready in Seattle." If participants want, they have the option of leaving the open chat room and going to a "private room" where they can have personal sexual conversations that may result in a face-to-face encounter.

Another area of acting out on the Internet involves reading or writing sexual fantasies. There are innumerable sites that contain graphic sexual fantasies. Some allow stories to be downloaded, and others facilitate posting of fantasies or swapping of stories. Worldwide, more than 100 million people visit pornographic websites monthly. However, this number is deceptively low. There is also a high percentage of peer-to-peer traffic offering pornographic materials that is not identified as visits to pornographic websites.

In addition, consider the intrusiveness of pornography in the pop-ups and spam emails reaching people who are innocently working on their computers. The pornography industry grabs tens of thousands of expired URLs each month and redirects people to active pornography sites. This so-called "porn-napping" has been experienced by many Internet users looking for a legitimate site who find a pornographic site instead.

Adults are not the only ones impacted by Internet pornography. The average age of first exposure to Internet pornography is eleven. One of the more recent practices among teens is the sending of text messages with attachments of nude or seminude photos of themselves to friends, known as "sexting." An alarming 20 percent of teens admit that they have been engaged in X-rated text messaging.[11]

Phone Sex

Phone sex lines predate the Internet. They are responsible for phone numbers with the 976 and 900 prefixes that automatically add toll charges to the phone bill of the caller. Although overt phone sex is illegal, loopholes allow the purveyors of the services to operate openly with little fear of prosecution. Charges for services range from a few cents to several dollars per minute. The typical use of phone sex is for the caller to tell his or her fantasy to the listener and then have the listener "talk dirty" while the caller masturbates. These numbers are frequently advertised in urban newspapers.

A New Spin on Voyeurism and Exhibitionism

Haden's Story

Haden was intrigued with miniature video cameras advertised online. He bought one, telling himself that he was going to use it for security in his home. Instead he installed it in his bathroom so he could secretly view overnight guests' behaviors. He then saved the videos on his computer. After he'd spent several months secretly recording videos of his friends, his daughter spotted something shiny in the vent in the bathroom. She told her mother, who discovered the camera. Incensed by what she found, she searched her husband's computer and found some of his videos. She took the computer to the police. After they found images of several young girls on his computer, Haden was arrested for possession of child pornography. He is now awaiting trial and has several additional charges pending.

The traditional image of a voyeur is the so-called "Peeping Tom" who lurks outside of bedroom windows hoping to see something tantalizing. However, consider what happened to this woman at a well-known hotel in a large city.

Veronica's Story

Veronica was in town for a business meeting. As was her usual morning routine, she went out for an early three-mile run and returned to her room to get ready for her meeting. Instead of turning on the light switch by the door of her darkened room, she walked across the room to turn on a lamp. Her eye was caught by a small beam of light on the mirror above the sink. She inspected the light more closely, and found that it was coming from behind the mirror. Putting her eye close to the mirror, Veronica could tell that the backing had been scraped away from the mirror, allowing her to see into a room behind the mirror.

Frightened by what she had found, she called the local police and told a detective what she discovered. The detective returned with her to the room and removed the mirror. A hole was revealed that led to a utility area that ran the entire length of the floor between adjacent rooms.

Hotel management was summoned to provide access to the utility area, and it was revealed that every room on that floor had a small peephole, allowing unrestricted viewing of the rooms. In the ensuing investigation, a maintenance man confessed that he had several webcams that he had set up in the space. He videotaped people in

*their rooms and also spent hours locked in the utility area, moving
from room to room to watch unsuspecting guests. While claiming this
was his first such encounter, he confessed that when he was a child he
used to watch his siblings through the bathroom door keyhole.*

While the incident may be an anomaly, it points out that we must
get beyond traditional stereotypes of sexual acting out. With the
advent of the Internet and inexpensive webcams, both voyeurism
and exhibitionism have been greatly facilitated. Misuse of webcams
is widespread. When a webcam is installed, the software often allows
the user to alert others online that a webcam is in use and enables a
link between the user and other webcams. This should be of special
concern to parents. Not only can children be targeted, but they may
be tempted to reenact juvenile "show me yours and I'll show you mine"
games with strangers.

Traditional Sites of Acting Out: Bookstores and Bathhouses

Hector's Story

*Hector recalls the shame he felt when he would have to shower after
gym class in school. He was sure his penis was much smaller than
those of the other boys. When he heard about pumps that would
enlarge his penis, he ordered one from an ad in a men's magazine.
The device did not work, so he searched for other devices. None of
the devices worked, but he got a degree of comfort believing that he
was a "late bloomer." He thought that he was just a bit behind other
boys and would eventually catch up.*

*By the time he got to college he realized that he would have to live
with the body parts he was born with. But Hector was not able to get
over his obsession with the size of his penis. While he believed that he
was heterosexual, he began acting out with men in the backrooms of
adult bookstores. Hector received affirmation from being with other
men, especially when he realized that many of them were not put*

off by his small size. He had tried to stop his acting out with men, believing it was a bad habit that he could control, but was unable to resist the urge to return to the same activities after making promises to himself that he would never repeat them.

Adult bookstores offer a variety of pornography and sometimes private booths where it is possible to view hard-core pornographic movies. These booths are usually dark and used for anonymous sexual encounters, primarily by men looking for sex with other men. They typically have "glory holes" in the wall of the adjoining booth that allow the participants to engage in anonymous sex without having to see the other person or to interact in any other way. Such bookstores are certainly dangerous, but some men feel so drawn to them that they find it nearly impossible to go more than a few days without visiting one.

Taamir's Story

Taamir moved to Chicago from the Middle East when he was fifteen. Having spent the first years of his life in a closed country, he had never seen pornography. Shortly after arriving in America he discovered that he could access pornography from any computer. He heard stories about what was available on the Internet but had never seen anything that was forbidden in his country. He was shocked with what he found, but soon his shock turned to fascination. By the time he was twenty, he spent every day either looking at pornography or trying to find someone who was willing to have sex with him. His meetings with acting-out partners became more frequent. Eventually he discovered bathhouses and soon was engaging in high-risk anonymous sexual behavior with as many partners as he could find.

The bathhouses referred to here exist in various large American and European cities, especially those with large gay populations. They are places where men hang out to have sex with other men. Often the goal is to have sex with as many men as possible.

Massage Parlors, Spas, Escort Services, and Related Businesses

Colin's Story

Colin's longtime partner, Sharon, experiences significant pain during intercourse. While she was working with her doctor to address her pain from a medical standpoint, Colin decided he would seek out the services of a massage parlor that offered a "happy ending" or would masturbate him for a "tip." He rationalized that he was not really cheating on his partner because he was not emotionally involved with anyone and had great love for Sharon. Besides, he was taking the pressure off Sharon to satisfy him sexually while she addressed her physical problems.

Gradually, Colin's trips to massage parlors increased to multiple times per week. He was no longer content with the manual stimulation he received but found that, for a price, he could engage in any sexual act. Ultimately he stopped the pretense that he was there for a massage and would just pay for sex. Colin tried to stop acting out but felt compelled to return to massage parlors to satisfy his addiction to sex. Results from a recent blood test revealed that he has a sexually transmitted disease. How is he going to explain this to Sharon?

Massage parlors set up to offer sex to their patrons should not to be confused with legitimate massage therapists. "Sexual" massage parlors are fronts for prostitution. They focus on selling sexual services and not on therapeutic massage. Commonly there are indications of their intent from how they market their services. These "sexual" massage parlors operate in many ways, but in the end the client always pays someone to perform sex.

Modeling studios and lingerie studios are another disguise for brothels that can be found in many large cities. Some require their patrons to pay a cover charge to enter and be allowed to watch women model various clothes or undergarments that they may want to purchase. These "studios" do not have anything to do with modeling clothing. They are other examples of houses of prostitution.

In some cities there are advertisements for photography studios. These supposedly allow photographers to find a model to pose nude. These studios will even rent cameras in case the customer does not have one, to give a greater appearance of legitimacy. But as with other sexual businesses, services offered behind closed doors provide more than just visual stimulation.

Escort services are plentiful and may even operate rather openly. They are advertised widely on the Internet. Do not believe the claims that these are just services that provide dates or social companions for lonely people. This is prostitution any way you look at it. The "escorts" pay a portion of their fee to their agency but make their real money on "tips," which are actually payment for sexual services. Patrons may pay a couple of hundred dollars or up to a thousand dollars or more for an "escort" and develop such an addiction to this behavior that they may even become convinced that they are in love with an escort they meet. Such misplaced emotions evolve because some of the time the escort will not charge or because the encounter may include long periods of talk as well as sex.

An old German expression says, "Be a lamb and the wolf shall appear." The same caution holds for sex addiction. Give in to your impulses and your addiction will take hold.

Our permissive society requires strong individual discipline, especially when it comes to sexual responsibility. It is not just the danger of contracting or passing on HIV or STDs that makes promiscuity damaging; it is the effect it has on the partner when the sex addict repeatedly and compulsively engages in self-indulgent forms of sexual behavior, creating lies and spreading deceit to conceal the addiction.

Just as someone addicted to substances sometimes needs to "hit bottom" to realize the seriousness of the problem, countless people addicted to sex need to experience a significant crisis before they will get into recovery. It could take exposure by a spouse, arrest by the police, termination by an employer, or the shame of being caught by family or friends for them to realize they are at the mercy of sex addiction.

Sex Addiction Among Physicians, Clergy, Senior Executives, and Celebrities

Sex addicts who are physicians, clergy, senior executives, and other high-salaried individuals or celebrities have much in common. They may perceive themselves as different from "ordinary" people. They may believe they live by a different set of rules than the rest of society. How do they justify this double standard? Simply because of the power they wield in their positions or the money they earn, which may be many times more than what ordinary people earn. All four groups have plentiful experiences reinforcing the belief that they are not like ordinary people.

Ravi's Story

A successful physician, Ravi enjoyed the finer things in life, but he did not get nearly as much pleasure from possessing nice things as he did from pursuing sex. A strip club near his office offered a "businessman's special," which was a lunch buffet for two dollars and a cover charge. Ravi developed the habit of eating at the club three days each week. He got to know the dancers by name and started dating one. He became interested in her when she told him she was working her way through medical school. In order for her to be able to afford to go out on a date, she needed him to cover the money she lost from tips by not working for the night. He was shocked to find out that she needed one thousand dollars to make up for lost tips for just one evening. Their relationship developed with them having a "date" once or twice a week. He eventually realized that her story about attending medical school was a lie. Before getting into recovery, Ravi realized that much of the money he had spent for the past year had been money he gave to his favorite dancer.

Society places physicians on a pedestal. Many people are raised not to challenge anything a physician says or does. As well-educated experts on health, physicians are respected, even revered by society.

In fairness to physicians, many do not seek this kind of attention and adulation. In fact, most go out of their way to present themselves as ordinary people who happen to be practicing the healing arts.

Yet hero worship prevails. Grateful patients and families of patients express their appreciation and tell physicians how they save lives. They may hear things like "You are the most gifted surgeon," or "Without you, I wouldn't be alive," or "Our town is fortunate to have you practicing here." Sincere comments may add to a physician's belief that he or she is not like ordinary people. The justification for acting out is a belief that they deserve a reward. They may feel they are due extra compensation for their long hours, unselfish devotion, and humanitarian efforts, or because they are so intelligent. Physicians may not have many relationships with people outside of their work, leading them to live isolated lives.

Keenan's Story

Keenan had wanted to be a minister since he was a teen. He also struggled with pornography at the same time. He would never think of violating his professional standards by beginning a sexual relationship with someone in his congregation. Because of his stature in his denomination, he is highly sought as a conference speaker and has a heavy travel schedule. On every trip Keenan scours the yellow pages and free press newspapers for spas and massage parlors. He is usually successful in finding someone willing to be sexual with him. While he feels guilty about his behavior, he reminds himself that he is helping many people through his ministry and that he is under extraordinary stress because of his busy schedule. He reasons that he deserves some relaxation and his sexual behavior is not harming anyone.

Clergy often work long hours for little pay. They may find they are always giving of themselves and seldom receiving. And as they perform their duties, there are frequently people who express their appreciation for many things a minister, priest, or rabbi does for them or their congregation. They may hear, "You're the best pastor we've ever had. God blessed us by sending you," or "No other rabbi has given so much of himself to the community." Most clergy do not seek to be put on a pedestal and do not ask to be idolized. But with the continued praise, some clergy may believe that they deserve a little something extra for their efforts.

As with all sex addicts, their acting-out behavior may include a wide variety of sexual activities. Sadly, physician and clergy acting out may include professional-boundary violations wherein they are involved sexually with patients, parishioners, or staff. Regardless of the behaviors involved, both physicians and clergy may be more isolated than other sex addicts and may find it more difficult to seek help for fear of being discovered.

Oliver's Story

Oliver had been the chief operating officer of a major corporation for nearly ten years. He was known as a "player" by his employees and had several consensual sexual relationships with various employees. His last affair with an employee began similarly to the others. It started with business lunches, followed by becoming sexual on out-of-town business trips. While he was not this person's direct supervisor, he knew he was jeopardizing his job by having sex with a subordinate.

Rumors began to circulate throughout the company as people speculated as to whether there was something more to his association with that particular employee than a work relationship. The employee was so embarrassed upon hearing the rumors that she finally went to the human resources department and confessed about the relationship. She feared getting fired for sleeping with the executive. Instead, the company launched an internal investigation and then confronted Oliver with the information. Oliver reluctantly admitted that he had had an affair with this person but pointed out that it had ended a month earlier, and that he never felt it compromised his job. He was dismissed by his company and was subsequently sued for sexual harassment. The six-figure settlement was borne partly by his company but mostly by Oliver. Worse yet was that other companies that might have been the source of future employment blackballed him from any position in his industry.

Some executives, entrepreneurs, and highly compensated individuals may believe their wealth and success separate them from the rest of society. They may see their success as evidence that they are unlike ordinary people. Their ability to be innovative and successful by going against conventional wisdom may reinforce their belief that they are not subject to the same rules and behavioral norms as the rest of society.

Because of their financial resources, there is a higher incidence of paying for sex among this population. One has only to look at the fall from power of various industry leaders and politicians to see the characteristics of individuals perceiving themselves to be above the rules and beyond the laws of society. Sex addicts who are senior executives may pay a significant amount of money for various sex partners. They may not see this as prostitution but instead believe they are helping out by providing living expenses and very extravagant gifts to their paramours. The greater the power, the greater the ability to rationalize one's behavior.

Money and access are extremely empowering to the executive addicted to sex who can escape detection for a long time with little repercussion. The wherewithal and the significant amount of travel involving hotels are particularly enabling. The sex trade that targets executives is found at all common business destinations including hotels and convention and conference centers, and is advertised and marketed with handout flyers and explicit in-room advertisements. Even hotel concierges, if asked, may provide numbers and contacts for escorts in the local sex trade.

Andy's Story

Andy recalls the first time he looked at pornography when he found a stash of magazines in a vacant apartment near his home. From his first look as a ten-year-old boy, he was hooked. He carefully guarded his treasure and hid it so that no one else could find it and take it from him. He began daily to sneak to this vacant apartment to look at the pictures. When he was not looking at the images, he was fantasizing about them.

In high school, Andy's natural athletic ability earned him a place on the varsity squad in several sports. His success, coupled with his good looks, garnered the attention of all the girls he craved. Throughout college he excelled in sports and became known as a womanizer, a reputation that continued into his professional life in sports. Andy moved from relationship to relationship with little more thought than he gave to changing sports cars—to have the newest and fastest. As far as anyone knew, Andy was successful in every area of life. But he knew he was incapable of stopping his acting out on his own. He never built a lasting relationship with anyone and felt lonely most of the time. To make matters worse, he realized his fame worked against him. He felt that it was impossible to get help for his addiction without having his private life exposed to the world on the network news.

We see the perks that come in the lives of celebrities. They may appear to have perfect lives. People are waiting on their every need and doors open to them because of their name or their reputation. They have financial resources great enough to fulfill any material desire. For those of us who have never been in the limelight, it may be hard to imagine the loneliness and isolation that can come with fame. Whether it is from the isolation that comes with renown or the aloofness sparked by thousands or millions of adoring fans, celebrities typically are not able to enjoy the things others take for granted.

For celebrities who find themselves addicted to problematic sexual behavior, they have the additional problem of not being able to embrace some of the recovery resources such as twelve-step groups, because their anonymity may be compromised. A few sex addiction treatment program professionals specialize in the particular needs of celebrity sex addicts.[12]

Treatment

Certain inpatient treatment programs cater to persons who are extremely well-known. One of the special challenges of inpatient treatment for this population is the occasional leaking of confidential information. What is intended to be private can end up in the tabloids.

There are twelve-step programs for people with sex addiction in communities all over the United States. Some locations offer twelve-step meetings for professionals. There are meetings specifically for clergy and physicians. These "specialty" meetings are helpful because people can benefit from being around those they can more easily identify with through shared professional experience in addition to their sex addiction.

Sex addiction is the great leveler. Ironically, the more power and money that go into maintaining the addiction, the greater the fall. Hitting bottom is the moment when the addict realizes he or she either must seek immediate help or lose everything. Sadly, numerous high-powered individuals, including physicians, clergy, executives, and celebrities, do not heed the message of hitting bottom because they believe their position, power, and/or affluence will provide permanent protection from the consequences of their actions. This is merely another facet of denial.

CHAPTER 3

UNSUCCESSFUL CURES

Jack's Story

Jack had always been successful. He took pride in the fact that he could spot business opportunities and turn them into successful ventures. His addiction to sex seemed to progress right along with his business acumen. Jack soon found that there were websites that were devoted to women who wanted to be taken care of by men.

He started meeting women he first contacted on "sugar daddy" sites and was relieved to find that he did not have to pay these women to have sex with him. He felt that they liked him because of who he was and for the special way he treated them. All of them would make requests from time to time that he help them with some of their financial needs. He would make mortgage payments, pay school tuition, purchase sports cars, and buy expensive jewelry for these women out of gratitude for the way they treated him. He kept an apartment near his office where he allowed one of his "sugar babies" to live.

Several times through the years, Jack realized how out of control his life had become. He made promises to himself that he was going to stop this behavior. One of his favorite promises was that he would stop his extracurricular relationships just as soon as he could figure out how to end his current affair. But as soon as one affair would end, he would go back to the sugar daddy websites and begin a new relationship. When Jack finally got into recovery, he calculated that he had spent several hundred thousand dollars on various women that he "kept." He strongly disagreed with his therapist, who said that these women were prostitutes. Jack said that they never charged him for having sex. They just accepted gifts he gave them.

Promises to Stop

What do people do to curb their problematic sexual behavior? They may try many things, and most of them are ineffective. One of the most common things people try is to make a promise that they will end their addictive behavior. They may make that promise to themselves, or, after being caught in their acting out, they may promise their spouse they will never go back to their harmful behavior. And for the most part, they are sincere in their promises. I encounter people who say they have made that promise to their spouse countless times in the past, and each time they meant it. However, they found they were not able to keep their promises.

Each New Year, addicts make resolutions that they will not go back to their old behavior. They are able to keep that resolution for a while, only to fall back into their old patterns. A variation of this is to swear an oath to God that one will put a permanent end to the problematic sexual behavior. This is especially true with those who are very religious or have a strong faith perspective. But each time they make that oath, they find they are unable to keep it.

The problem is not the sincerity of the person making the promise or oath or a lack of power on the part of God. The problem is that there is an addiction present that must receive specific treatment in order for there to be success. Each time a person is unable to keep a promise or fulfill an oath, his or her self-esteem plummets and the sense of hopelessness increases.

Become More Religious

Some sex addicts believe that the reason they act out is because they have not prayed correctly or have not followed a particular tenet of their faith. They may feel they have not attended services often enough or read the Bible or other sacred text enough. They may believe they are just not committed enough to God.

So their solution is to become more religious. They attend services more frequently. They commit themselves to various spiritual disciplines. They commit to reading the Bible cover to cover, give more money to their religion, and generally become more focused on spiritual matters. While all of these things are good and have the potential to be helpful, they do not cure addiction in any of its forms, including sex. And when the acting out returns, that person has his or her original ideas reinforced—that he or she indeed is not committed enough and does not love God enough.

Geographical Cure

There are people who think that perhaps the problem is the area in which they live. On the surface it may seem that the thing to do is to get a complete change of environment. The place where you live may have many acting-out opportunities. Perhaps living in an area with less temptation would help you be more successful in recovery.

A variation of this is to get a different job or live in a different house. Certainly there are changes in environment that can be made that will help a person be more successful in recovery. But just changing locations will not put an end to acting out. When people are caught up in addictive behavior they are compelled to repeat it, and wherever they are they will find outlets for it. Geographical cures simply do not work. Among other realities, the Internet is everywhere.

Get into a Relationship or Get Married

Single people may look at their life and think the solution to their sexual acting out is to get into a relationship or to get married. They reason that if they are married there would not be any need to act out. They would have a willing sex partner always available, and that would keep them from acting out. However, there are numerous married men whose spouse is willing to be sexual with them but who still choose to act out with other partners. Clearly the availability of a sex partner is not enough to stem the tide of acting out. In fact, many partners of sex addicts have said that there is very little sex taking place in their relationship. They may even be shocked to find out they are married to a sex addict, because that person seldom wanted to have sex with them.

Get a Divorce or End a Relationship

Conversely, some married sex addicts believe that their problem would be solved if they could just get out of their current relationship. They believe the reason they act out is because they are not married to the right person. They may think that if they could just get free from their current relationship, they would then be able to find the "right" person to marry and that would solve everything. Unfortunately, people have tried this only to find out that their addiction was not cured by ending their relationship. They just went on to another relationship and found that their desire to act out continued.

Cure It with a Pill

Some sex addicts have sought out the care of a physician in the hope of ending their acting out. They reason that there must be some medication that will take away their obsessive desire for sex. Some have sought out hormone treatment to lower their sex drive. Others have operated on the premise that if they addressed other mental or emotional concerns, their sex addiction would be cured in the process.

Certainly there are medications that lower sex drive. Some physicians even prescribe these with the hope of ending a person's acting out. But sex addiction is not the result of having too strong a sex drive. Sex addiction develops due to a number of factors. A lower sex drive may support other recovery efforts but will not by itself cure sex addiction. Medications that are needed to treat other co-occurring disorders such as depression, ADHD, and other mental or emotional disorders are very helpful in recovery. But sex addiction cannot be cured by taking any pill. Since sex addiction is both a thought disorder and a behavioral disorder, persons hoping to recover from sex addiction must change their patterns of thinking and acting, and consider twelve-step recovery approaches—twelve-step meetings, working with a sponsor, and working through the Twelve Steps of recovery.

Outgrow the Addiction

Some believe that they will just outgrow their addiction. They feel that as part of the natural aging process they will outlast their obsessive thinking and compulsive actions. But I have had a number of clients in their seventies who are still acting out. I have had a few clients in their eighties who still battle addiction to sex. Recently a man told me that the police called him and asked him to go to the jail to pick up his father, who was in his mid-nineties. The man was picked up when he was acting out inside an adult video store. You will not live long enough to outlive sex addiction.

Nip and Tuck

Some female partners believe that they can curb their partner's sexual acting-out behavior by getting plastic surgery. They reason that if they had a more perfect body, there would be no reason for their partner to act out. Some women have had multiple cosmetic procedures for this purpose. But the problem is not with the looks of the partner. The problem is with the sex addict. I have known women who have won major beauty contests whose husbands act out with other women. Their husbands are sex addicts. They are not seeking beauty. They are pursuing an addiction that is never satisfied and destroys everything that is good and precious.

If you are the partner of a sex addict and you are considering plastic surgery, first ask yourself if you are doing it in an effort to change the behavior of your partner. Wanting surgery for your own reasons (to help you feel more attractive or to correct some significant flaw or defect) is understandable. But if you are doing it to change your partner's behavior, think again before proceeding. He will not stop his acting-out behavior just because you change your looks.

Lingerie Cure

There are female partners who believe that the way to keep their partners from acting out is to get new lingerie. They may spend great sums of money on lingerie that they hope will help them become more sexually desirable. But most are disappointed to find out that the new lingerie does not make a difference. In fact, some women take a significant hit to their self-esteem when they find that even the latest Paris boudoir collection is ineffective in stopping their husband's acting out.

Bedroom Gymnastics

Through the years some uninformed therapists and counselors and a number of misguided clergy, as well as some widely read books, have encouraged women to be more sexual and more sexually creative in order to bring an end to their partner's acting out. The thinking is that since the problem is sexual in nature, more and/or different sex is the answer. But bedroom gymnastics will not cure sexual acting out.

Whatever a couple determines to do as part of their sexuality (as long as other people or pornography are not involved and as long as it is not hurtful, demeaning, or degrading) is up to that couple. They do not need anyone else to give them permission for what they do within the confines of their bedroom. But partners of sex addicts need to be clear that they will not be able to stop their partner's acting out by stretching themselves sexually.

Other Things That Do Not Work

There are other things that do not work in eradicating sex addiction. For example, worry will not put an end to sex addiction. Neither will self-pity. "Rule keeping" will not alleviate sex addiction. This is not to be confused with setting healthy boundaries; rather, it is having a system of rigid rules to follow in the belief they will keep someone from acting out. Hoping, wishing, and having good intentions will not keep a person from acting out sexually. The only thing that works in treating sex addition is embarking on a recovery journey that is neither an easy path nor one that provides a quick resolution.

Sex addiction is a formidable foe that is not easily stamped out. But it is possible to put an end to all acting-out behaviors. If you are willing to work hard and stop trying to develop your own cure, you can find freedom from destructive addictive sexual behaviors. Keep reading. You are on the right course.

CHAPTER 4

ADDRESSED TO THE SEX ADDICT

Stan's Story

Stan has been dressing up like a woman for years. He doesn't recall the first time, but remembers when he found a discarded pair of his mother's pantyhose when he was about seven or eight and tried them on to see what he looked like. When he was a teen, Stan was dressing up in his mother's clothes whenever she was away.

Stan felt most free to act out when he traveled out of town on business. He liked to dress up as a woman and then find anonymous men for brief sexual encounters. He frequently shipped company supplies ahead in preparation for a business meeting, and would regularly pack his dress-up clothes with the company supplies. The boxes were shipped to his hotel with a note that they were to be opened only by him. This allowed him to travel with only a carry-on piece of luggage and reduced the possibility that his wife would discover his secret behavior.

On one trip, his flight was delayed by weather, causing him to arrive a day late. He was not concerned, because he would still be there in time to unpack his box and hide his female wardrobe and complete preparations for the scheduled business meeting. What he did not know was that his boss had arrived a day earlier than scheduled. His boss retrieved the supply box from the hotel and unpacked it to prepare for the meeting. Imagine his surprise when he found women's clothes in the company supply box, complete with a photo of Stan in his Sunday best! The next week Stan was busy searching the Internet for treatment for his sex addiction.

The Crisis

The crisis that brought you to recovery is the proverbial blessing in disguise. That crisis may be the threat of loss or the actual loss of a relationship, job, health, or freedom. As painful as it is, if the crisis leads you into recovery, it can be the best thing that has ever happened to you.

I have heard confessions of years of acting out. I have also listened as individuals revealed acting out that began only recently. Partners have said they turned on their computer and found a secret email their partner wrote to a lover. A man had finished a cell phone conversation with his wife and then propositioned a prostitute, and later learned his spouse overheard the entire episode because he forgot to press "end" to finish the phone call. One woman became addicted to problematic sexual behavior concealed behind the fantasy of an avatar on an Internet site.

Guys often fall into the trap of being the knight in shining armor. They want to rescue others—particularly women. They may intentionally seek out needy women so they can receive gratitude when they solve their problems. For some, it is solving a financial problem. The sex addict may think he can afford it and think little of providing monetary support. But that is the beginning of the journey into addictive behavior. Or maybe a guy just wants to comfort and support a coworker who is having a difficult time. Twelve-step rooms are filled with guys who "just wanted to help" but ended up in a relationship with someone who was not their partner. They claim not to know how they got there. But they got there because they set out to rescue some vulnerable and needy person.

Often the crisis is difficult to face. But if crisis leads to recovery and changes how you live, it can be a turning point for you to move forward. Since you are reading this book, you know there is no longer a chance of things remaining the same. Even the crisis of losing a job or being arrested may be seen as a gift because it can be the beginning of the road to recovery. I ask that you try your very best to adhere to the message and the methods of hope and freedom described in this book for you and your partner.

Hope and Freedom for Both of You

For your relationship to be restored, you—the sex addict—and your partner must ultimately commit to the difficult but rewarding journey called recovery. The paths each of you take may be different, but the goal of healing and of having a healthy relationship is the same.

Though it may seem unfair, your partner will need to be involved in his or her own recovery, even though you have the addiction. Your addiction has greatly impacted the person you love.

You may have tried numerous "cures" throughout the years and believe that you are beyond help. All sex addicts hope to become truly content and not go outside the boundaries of their marriages or loving primary relationships. As unbelievable as it may seem, your acting out can come to an end. There is hope that you will finally follow through on your commitment to be faithful to your partner. This may seem like an impossible dream, but I have seen this dream come true many times.

- Recovery means an end to seeking sex outside of the marriage/ primary relationship.

- Recovery means the end to concealment and deceit.

- Recovery means hope for you to become a person of integrity.

- There is no time but *now* and there is no place but *here*.

Immediate Steps Toward Hope and Freedom[13]

End problematic relationships. The first action for sex addicts is to terminate all contact with acting-out partners. This means contacting each of them and explicitly stating that the relationship is over and there will be no further contact. This contact should be done under the supervision of a trusted friend, sponsor, or therapist.

Change cell phone number and email address. These actions are necessary whenever there has been sexual acting out with others who have this contact information. It is imperative for sex addicts to change their email address and cell phone number immediately. I get more resistance from my sex-addicted clients about this action than any other. I hear what a nuisance it is or how impossible it will be for them to make these changes. These changes may be inconvenient, but sex addiction is a disorder that causes many unpleasant things to occur. Recovery can make great improvements in your quality of life, but it is a process that requires making significant changes.

Getting a new cell phone number and email address are necessary if there is even one acting-out partner who knows how to contact you. Also, it is important to resign immediately from all social networks. If there were *any* contacts through company email, you should consult the company's human resources department and ask if it is possible to get a new email address. If your cell phone is provided by the company, you may need to consult with human resources for help in getting a new phone number assigned. These changes may create some difficulty with your company, but they are necessary to help you break free from your addiction.

I am often told how this will not be necessary because "everyone knows I'm in recovery and they are not to call me anymore." I also hear about how this is not necessary since several weeks or even months have passed since there was any contact with an acting-out partner. But leaving the possibility open for a former partner to contact you is inviting a slip or relapse. If a former partner calls and you are not in a strong place, the chances of giving in to sexual impulses and engaging in acting-out behavior are great. Even if you are in a strong place in your recovery, you will need to tell your spouse about this contact, and that will surely add tension and stress to a relationship that is already strained.

End all secret accounts. The first day of recovery should also be spent closing all "extra" email accounts, getting rid of secret cell phones, closing any secret post office boxes as well as any secret bank and credit card accounts, and closing secret bank safe-deposit boxes. The web of deceit and deception must be completely eliminated. The best time to make the most significant gains in changing behavior is at the beginning of recovery.

Delete all screen names and profiles. Screen names that were used for acting out should be eliminated from all computers you have used. This will involve cleaning all of the "cookies" off the computer or wiping the computer clean of all identifiers. Any "handle" that was used in a chat room and any profiles that were used in chat rooms or dating services should be erased. The recovering addict must not return to any of the haunts of his or her addictive behavior, be they real or virtual.

Trash the "little black book." Permanently destroy all contact information from former acting-out partners. Do not keep a backup list. Eliminate this contact information from all computers, mobile devices, and printed address books.

Dump the pornography "stash." Any stash of pornography must be disposed of immediately. If you have videos or DVDs hidden in your home or office, a thorough search must be made to make sure all of them are found and discarded. This should be done under the supervision of a trusted friend, accountability partner, sponsor, or someone from a twelve-step group. It is also necessary to have the hard drive of your computers professionally "cleaned" to remove all traces of past acting-out behavior. However, if you have ever accessed underage pornography, you would be better off destroying your hard drive rather than risk getting it serviced by a computer repair facility.

Make a commitment to recovery. The first day in recovery is also a day to make a commitment to stay in recovery and do *whatever it takes* to be free from acting out. This commitment will have to be solidified on a daily basis throughout your recovery process. From the very beginning, sex addicts need to make a commitment to themselves that they will be ruthless in their pursuit of recovery.

Consult with a psychiatrist or other behavioral health professional. Early in the recovery process I believe it is useful for the recovering addict to be evaluated by a psychiatrist to see if there are other disorders present that need to be treated in order to successfully address the sex addiction. Mood disorders, including anxiety and depression, attention deficit hyperactivity disorder (ADHD), and other disorders are frequently present with sex addiction. These may need to be managed through medication. If any of these disorders are present and are not effectively managed as part of an overall recovery strategy, it will be much more difficult, if not virtually impossible, for sex addicts to successfully stop their acting out.

Read about sex addiction. From the start of recovery, sex addicts should develop a habit of reading all they can about sex addiction and recovery. Reading this book is a good start. You must become knowledgeable about the addiction that has so devastated your life. At the end of this book, you will find an extensive bibliography along with websites and addresses of agencies and organizations dedicated to overcoming sex addiction.

Develop daily spiritual disciplines. Without help from a Higher Power, as it is referred to in twelve-step programs, or, as many people prefer, God, I believe it is impossible for a person to end all acting out and live in continued recovery. I know many disagree with this and believe that an individual can "pick himself up by his own bootstraps." The members of twelve-step fellowships recognize the importance of calling on God or a Higher Power to help do for them what they cannot alone do for themselves. Each individual is free to believe in the Higher Power of his or her choice. In terms of recovery from addiction, what matters is not whether you are Christian, Jew, Muslim, Hindu, or a member of any other religion or sect, but that you recognize there is something greater than you that can be accessed to lead you out of the darkness of addiction and into the light of recovery.

Develop daily physical disciplines. Two important disciplines in successful recovery are getting regular sleep and daily exercise. Sleep should last for a minimum of seven hours per night and preferably eight hours. Often sex addicts do not get enough sleep because they spend so many late evening hours acting out on the Internet or watching movies after the rest of the family is in bed. If there is a history of insomnia, it may be advisable to see one's physician to address the sleep problems. In some cases a "sleep study" may be indicated to help restore a normal pattern and level of sleep. There are other physical disciplines that should also be cultivated, such as maintaining a healthy diet, regular dental checkups, and annual physical exams. When persons are active in their addiction, they may neglect these important disciplines—either because their acting out is taking so much of their time or because they fail to think about their physical health and personal appearance.

Avoid certain things. All substances that were used in connection with sexual acting out need to be reviewed and, if possible, eliminated from one's lifestyle. Healthy living dictates the elimination of tobacco in any form. Caffeine is a stimulant that it is prudent to curtail or eliminate from one's diet. Alcohol should also be limited or eliminated. Illegal drug use should be ended, and prescription medication that is taken on a routine basis should be scrutinized. Is the medication still needed? Can it be eliminated without health repercussions? Your physician should help you make decisions regarding prescription medications.

Establish work-related boundaries. Recovery may mean an immediate change in one's daily work routine. Some people are working with former acting-out partners. The ultimate solution to this very uncomfortable situation may be to change jobs. Others have crossed boundaries with some employees that need to be reestablished at the beginning of recovery.

Another boundary surrounding one's career has to do with the number of hours worked. Is it necessary to work as many hours as usual? Some people may observe some workaholic behaviors that need to be addressed. A point comes when a person crosses the line from being a conscientious employee to being obsessed with work performance.

Become a careful consumer of media. Sex addicts find that they need to be careful about what they allow to come into their minds through the media. Certainly there are suggestive movies and TV shows you will not want to watch. This is not because someone else is scrutinizing your viewing habits, but because you are acknowledging that certain media/entertainment content is a threat to your sexual sobriety.

For some recovering sex addicts, this means no longer listening to a particular type of music. For others, this means there are certain songs that they choose not to listen to. This decision is especially relevant if certain music was used when acting out or even in the rituals leading up to acting out. Some cities have a "free press" newspaper that contains interesting articles. However, some of them also print so-called adult services ads used by sex addicts for locating their preferred acting-out arrangement. In such cases, addicts must protect themselves by simply having a personal boundary of not reading those publications.

Have fun. In the midst of recovery, life may take on a somber tone. Recovery is certainly serious business that requires many hours of work each week. That doesn't mean people can't relax and have fun. If anything, the recovering addict will find that life free of addiction is rich with discovery.

CHAPTER 5

ADDRESSED TO THE PARTNER

Cynthia's Story

Cynthia married Hershel four years ago. Their marriage has not been perfect, but it has been satisfying for both. As far as she knew, Hershel had been faithful to her. But when she went to the doctor for her gynecological exam, she discovered she had contracted a sexually transmitted disease. She had not been with anyone but Hershel and got a clean bill of health on previous exams. She confronted Hershel when he got home from work. He vigorously denied any sexual involvement with anyone else and became incensed by the accusations. But over the next several weeks, Cynthia found evidence on his computer that Hershel was corresponding with multiple people for sexual liaisons. When he realized he could no longer deny his behavior, Hershel admitted having a long-term sexual addiction that involved high-risk sexual behavior with men and women, most of whom were strangers.

Why Does the Sex Addict Do It?

When you discovered your partner's problematic sexual behavior, you probably asked many "why" questions. Why does he or she do those things? Why can't he or she be satisfied with me? Why doesn't my partner love me enough to stop this behavior?

On top of these questions are other questions. What did I do to cause this? How did I fail my spouse? Did this happen because I am not pretty or handsome enough? Did I cause this by not being more sexual with my partner? How can I get him or her to stop acting out? Is there any hope for our relationship? How can I be sure he or she doesn't go back to this behavior in the future?

This chapter covers these and other questions. It addresses why the sex addict continues the compulsive behavior. This is an especially troubling question if you have caught your spouse acting out in the past and he or she promised to stop. The short answer is that the problematic sexual behavior continues because he or she is addicted.

A lot of misinformation about sex addiction persists. One misunderstanding some people have is that when people say they are sex addicts, they are freed from responsibility for their actions. This is not true. The diagnosis of sex addiction helps explain why a person will risk losing so much to pursue sexual activity. But sex addicts remain totally responsible for their actions. The addict's best action is to have boundaries around certain behaviors in which they will not participate.

Another misconception about sex addiction is that all sex addicts are "perverts." The typical sex addict today may or may not be involved in viewing Internet pornography and compulsive masturbation. They may or may not be involved in sexual behavior with other people. And their behavior may or may not include any number of hundreds of specific sexual behaviors that others would consider "perverted."

Rebecca's Story

Rebecca discovered her husband's acting out when he left his computer on with his email open. There were numerous pornographic emails he had received from various women. Rebecca found that most of the emails were responses to sexual emails that had been sent by her husband. She was devastated by this discovery. The question she continued to ask herself was why her husband had gone somewhere else for his sexual fulfillment. She was sure it had something to do with her. Wondering what she did to deserve the hurt her husband had caused, she sought the services of a therapist. The therapist suggested that it might be helpful if she got some new lingerie and became a bit more adventurous in the bedroom. This furthered Rebecca's belief that her husband's acting out was her fault.

This therapist's suggestion was not only completely wrong, it was harmful to Rebecca. In truth, Rebecca was not at fault for her husband's acting out. She did not cause it, and nothing she did could change his behavior. Her husband made the choice to act out, and it was not the result of anything Rebecca did or did not do. Unfortunately, the misguided suggestion by Rebecca's therapist is not an isolated case. Counseling professionals who do not have expertise in treating sex addiction may make the erroneous suggestion that changing the partner's behavior will cause the unwanted sexual behaviors to stop. Nothing could be further from the truth.

It Is Not Your Fault

Perhaps you have asked yourself why your spouse is not satisfied with you or how you have failed to satisfy his or her desires. What have you done that has caused your partner to seek other sexual outlets?

The answer is that his or her behavior is not your fault. You did not cause it. Nothing you said or did resulted in your partner becoming caught up in this form of addiction. That may be hard to accept, especially if your partner has reminded you of a fight that the two of you had or of a cruel remark you made. Sex addicts may point to such situations, which they manufacture to provide them with an excuse to act out, as the "reason" that they sought sex outside of your relationship.

There may be many factors that contribute to a person's decision to act out sexually. And there may even be traumatic events that happened, particularly in childhood, that helped shape the decisions he or she made. But sex addicts have to take responsibility for their own decisions and their own actions, and the subsequent consequences. Accepting responsibility for their actions is at the heart of the work of recovery. You did not cause the addiction, even if you look at your life and believe there are extenuating circumstances that may have contributed to your spouse's behavior.

Your partner is responsible for his or her behavior and cannot avoid responsibility by complaints like "He just doesn't understand me" or "She doesn't want to have sex as often as I do." Your partner chose to get involved in sexual behavior that has now become compulsive and is very destructive to your relationship. There are many things that may contribute to a person's choice to act out, but the bottom line is that your partner made that choice to act out. You are not responsible for it, but you can take charge of how you are going to respond to it. If you have been told that you caused the sex addict's behavior, take solace in the fact that he or she made the decision to act out and it is his or her responsibility.

How Then Can You Get Your Partner to Stop Acting Out Sexually?

Just as you did not cause his or her addiction, you cannot control it or cure it. There is nothing you can do to stop the behavior. However, you can take care of yourself and decide that you are going to get healthy. You can also insist that the only way you will continue in the relationship is if your partner stops acting out immediately and engages in a program of recovery. You will need help in establishing and maintaining these boundaries. Having clear and healthy boundaries is essential for your individual well-being, as well as for the two of you if you and your partner are to have any chance for a healthy and lasting relationship.

Some individuals enter recovery because they know it is the only opportunity they have to save the relationship. For their recovery to be successful, they will have to shift their focus. When a person gets to the point where he or she is willing to do whatever it takes to get free from problematic sexual behavior, whether the relationship survives or not, then the addict is at a place where recovery has the greatest chance of success. Establishing new boundaries of what is acceptable and what is unacceptable to you may help your partner make the first important move toward recovery.

You may be wondering if your relationship has any hope of surviving. Things may look very bleak, especially as you learn the sordid details of your partner's behavior. The good news is that there is hope for your relationship not only to survive but even to thrive *if* your partner commits to recovery, and *if* both of you determine that you are willing to do whatever is necessary for your relationship to be restored.

Some people are not willing to do the work necessary for the relationship to flourish. They look at the pain they have already endured and decide they have had enough, and it is just easier to end the relationship. When faced with trauma, they want the pain to stop, and the easiest way to do that is by ending the relationship. Yet even if they do end the relationship, there is still work that both partners will need to do if they are going to be able to be successful in future relationships. Recovery is worth the effort. When a sex addict is painstaking about achieving recovery and the significant other in his or her life is willing to help work on the issues together, they can achieve a new trust and reciprocal respect unknown to couples whose relationship has never been fundamentally tested.

If My Partner Is a Sex Addict, Why Isn't He or She More Sexual with Me?

One reason sex addicts do not have sex as often with their spouses is because their acting out drains energy from the relationship and they need the neurochemical high they get from a new or forbidden relationship or secret behavior. They are sexual with other people or they masturbate compulsively, and that literally drains their energy and lessens any sexual desire they have toward their partner.

Some sex addicts are never sexual with other people but confine their acting out to viewing pornography, engaging in sexual cyberchat, or phone sex. And with many of these behaviors, there is often also compulsive masturbation. A male sex addict may say, "My wife thinks I have been unfaithful, but all I do is look at pornography and masturbate." From his perspective, he believes he has been faithful. But from the wife's perspective, she sees him as unfaithful because he is choosing to be sexual with pictures of people (or to have sexual chats or phone sex) rather than to be sexual with her.

It is true that men and women may view sexual behavior around pornography, sexual chat rooms, or phone sex differently. Some men want to adopt a definition of infidelity that includes only intercourse with someone other than their spouse. And thanks in part to memorable comments by a national politician about oral sex, these men want to convince others that only intercourse qualifies as fitting the definition of "having sex." But their female partners often view any sex outside of their exclusive relationship as being unfaithful. The male sex addict mistakenly thinks, "She doesn't understand that looking at pornography and masturbation are harmless."

Perhaps you have thought there must be something wrong with you if your husband or wife is having sex outside of your marriage and having little or no sex with you. Perhaps you have even been told that the reason your partner is sexual outside of your relationship is because you are not sexy enough, you complain too much, or in some other way the focus and blame for his or her behavior is shifted to you. This is classic "blame game" behavior for sex addicts. They convince themselves that they are not responsible for their behavior but are victims of a bad marriage, an unloving spouse, a stressful job, or any of hundreds of other excuses.

Even if the sex addict finds a partner whose sexual appetites are similar to his or her own, continued sex with the same person over a period of time results in more normalized neurochemical levels. What some call the "adrenaline rush" (or, more accurately, an increased level of dopamine, norepinephrine, and a variety of other neurotransmitters as well as cortisol) diminishes. The lower level of neurochemical reinforcement does not satisfy people who become addicted to sex. While they are now married and have a willing partner for sexual fulfillment, they are not satisfied. They look for other partners or for other means of securing higher neurochemical levels in their brain, such as engaging in high-risk sex or engaging in sexual practices that are degrading, dehumanizing, or illegal.

Frequently, sex addicts who are married to partners who normally have very high sex drives opt for such a low level of sexual activity that weeks or even months will pass without any desire for sex. In a number of cases, I have known of otherwise healthy, young individuals forgoing sex with their partner for years, choosing instead to satisfy their sexual needs with problematic sexual behavior outside of what the partner thought was a committed relationship. They look for other sex partners and often get as much of the rush they are seeking out of the pursuit as they do out of the sexual activity that appears to be their goal.

Why Do They Continue to Pursue Other Avenues of Sexual Expression When It Appears They Have All That They Could Ask for Waiting at Home?

The answer to this question is that the goal of their sexual activities is not intercourse or even physical sexual release, but rather a neurochemical fix. Some married sex addicts believe the way for them to stop acting out is to find a partner who will "love me as I deserve, give me sex any time I want it, and not nag me about doing things around the house." In short, they have the emotional maturity of adolescents who want to have all of the fun that life has to offer without assuming any of the responsibilities. Whether they are married or not, and regardless of whether their partner has a high sex drive or a more normal or even low sex drive, they will continue to seek to get high by engaging in one or several of a wide variety of sexual activities. Again, the goal is not sex but rather to get their "fix."

Is He or She a Narcissist?

Sex addicts are selfish—very selfish. They want what they want, when they want it. They may be more concerned about what makes them feel good or loved, or what makes them feel lonely, than they are about others. Even for sex addicts who are outwardly gentle, seemingly caring persons, inwardly they place their desires ahead of those of their partner and everyone else. Rather than being concerned about being faithful to their partner, sex addicts see their own desire to fulfill their selfish cravings as paramount.

Sex addicts can be manipulative. They may be able to cry on demand in order to make themselves more believable or to elicit sympathy. They may wear their feelings on their sleeve and claim that they are just sensitive. However, this behavior is very often attention-seeking and manipulative. Rather than being sensitive, for many sex addicts this is just another manifestation of narcissism.

Since sex addicts are typically narcissistic, does that make them pathologically narcissistic? In other words, do they meet the clinical criteria for narcissistic personality disorder, or NPD? Fortunately, that is not usually the case. NPD is present in less than 1 percent of the general population, according to the *Diagnostic and Statistical Manual of Mental Disorders (DSM)*.[14] This is an important truth to hear because there are plenty of either poorly informed persons or perhaps badly wounded partners who speak out on the Internet and other forums, trying to make the case that most sex addicts have NPD. Although the extreme self-centeredness driven by active sex addiction does mimic the symptoms of narcissistic personality disorder, when the addict achieves stable recovery those symptoms usually decrease significantly.

Compulsive Masturbation

Maurice's Story

Maurice had never been sexual with anyone other than his wife. Raised in a very conservative family, Maurice did not date much as a teenager. With his family's very strict religious beliefs, he did not feel he was allowed to ask questions about sex or have any real sex education. His parents did have "the talk" with him when he was fifteen. His father told him that when he was married, he would get very close to his wife and that their resulting relationship would produce babies.

More confused than informed, he found some sex education from friends. To further fill the information void, Maurice started looking up sexual topics on the Internet. He found that he could get information on any sexual behavior and could even find photos and videos of people engaging in various sexual acts. That early search for knowledge turned into a time-consuming addiction by the time he was married. When his wife finally caught him looking at pornography online, he had developed a habit of engaging in cybersex behaviors for at least two hours a day. Most of his behavior was limited to browsing pornographic websites, but he recently has been following conversations in sexual chat rooms.

While he has not yet engaged in chat with anyone, Maurice is thinking about starting what he considers to be harmless chat. While online he has masturbated, sometimes multiple times a day. A few times he masturbated to the point of injury. Lately, Maurice's wife has complained that he is just not interested in sex with her, and she wonders why not. He realizes that he needs to stop this behavior because of the negative impact it is having on his marriage. But so far he has not been successful in being able to stop his compulsive masturbation or his use of online pornography.

The topic of masturbation is difficult for some people to talk about. Studies show that virtually all men and a significant portion of women have masturbated at one time or another. There is an assumption that masturbation is something individuals outgrow as they leave their teenage years. In fact, a number of people, both men and women, continue masturbating throughout their adult lives. Masturbation not only can have a negative impact on the sexual relationship in committed relationships, but it may also impact communication and conflict-resolution skills.

How Can Masturbation Damage a Relationship Outside of the Sexual Realm?

The answer is that women and men approach sex differently. Women typically require an emotional connection with their partner if they are going to have sex. If problems or conflict exist in the relationship, they must be addressed before many women are willing to be sexual. It is a different story with men. Men do not have to have an emotional connection to have sex. They can completely separate sex from love or emotion. If a man wants to be sexual but there is some emotional baggage in the relationship, his wife will probably want to "unpack" that baggage before being sexual. As for him, if he is not willing to wait or make the emotional investment in the relationship, he can masturbate—literally be sexual with himself—and not have to expend any emotional energy.

The fact is that sexually addicted men may choose to continue their self-centered, narcissistic acting out through masturbation rather than attend to the emotional and communication concerns of the relationship. For many men, masturbation becomes a compulsive act that they use to medicate pain, stress, loneliness, fear, anger, or other emotions. For that reason, I believe that masturbation within a committed relationship is often selfish and may contribute significantly to the couple having a lower-than-desired frequency of sexual intimacy.

Perhaps the biggest problem with masturbation is that it is a gateway behavior that often ignites other acting-out behaviors. Before frequenting sexual massage parlors, before the clandestine affair, before seeking out prostitutes, many sex addicts have spent numerous sessions masturbating and then rationalizing their behavior by saying that they were engaging only in masturbation and fantasy. In other words, they see the self-gratifying action as pertaining only to themselves and not to their spouse as a statement of rejection or withholding of pleasure. The neurochemical reinforcement provided when one masturbates to fantasy is powerful. The resulting changes in brain chemistry give a person a high not unlike the high that comes from using certain illegal drugs.

Promises, Lies, and More Promises

You caught him or her looking at pornography several times. Each time, your partner has made promises to stop and never do it again. Or you found out your partner had an affair (or perhaps repeated affairs). Again, promises were made that the affair(s) would end, but you have evidence that it is (they are) still going on. What do you do? Will you ever be able to trust your partner again? That is the question that nags at the core of your being. You want to trust the person you love, but you have found that there is a web of deception between the two of you, and you wonder if your partner will ever be truthful with you.

I tell the partners of sex addicts that a person cannot be successful as a sex addict without being a world-class liar. This is not a character assassination but a statement of fact. A sex addict lies not only to cover up acting out, but to preserve the image of him- or herself that the unsuspecting world holds. Sex addicts believe—not without validity— that if their partner knew about everything they had done in the past as well about as their current acting-out behaviors, he or she would not stay in the relationship.

Sex addicts will often lie not only about their problematic sexual behavior, but also about some small and seemingly meaningless things. When asked questions concerning why they were late, what happened to a broken flowerpot, or other relatively unimportant questions, addicts may lie.

Why Does He or She Lie (Even About Little Things)?

Lying may be the toughest habit for your partner to break. For some sex addicts, even after they have stopped acting out and have started doing significant work in recovery, lying can be a difficult habit to discontinue. For example, if you ask your partner if he remembered to put out the trash, he might lie and tell you that he did, even though he did not. In his mind he may rationalize that he can get it taken care of before you get home, so it really does not count as a lie.

Why do people lie? Initially, lying may develop as a survival skill. If a child has a parent who is abusive and perhaps caught up in his or her own addiction, a child may lie to keep from being abused. Or, if a child is neglected, ignored, or in some other way marginalized, he or she may lie to get attention. Sometimes children with a learning disability or another limiting factor may lie to appear more normal. Lying learned in childhood is often difficult to stop, having become ingrained and carried into adulthood.

People may lie as self-defense. They shade the truth to make themselves appear in a better light. Some people invent a web of deception to make themselves appear more interesting or more successful in the hope it will make people like them more. Partners wonder how far the lying extends. "If she lied when she said she was on a business trip, how do I know she is not lying when she says she loves me?" After the first revelation of acting out, partners find that their familiar world begins to come apart. The person they thought they could trust has not only been lying but has been involved in sexual behavior that has shattered that trust.

Discussed in a later chapter, polygraph exams can be useful tools for helping a sex addict cultivate the habit of telling the truth, as long as they are used as an integrated part of therapy with a skilled sex addiction therapist. Sticking to a regular schedule of follow-up exams after a formal disclosure can be an integral part of therapy, and reinforces the habit of living within the truth. As the sex addict continues in recovery, he or she will come to recognize the invaluable necessity of truth-telling skills, even if that necessity is imposed by the partner as a condition for not leaving the marriage or relationship.

Is It My Fault?

Your partner may have told you repeatedly that his or her acting out is entirely your fault. He or she may have said unkind things to you including that you are not attractive to him or her, that he or she does not love you (perhaps never has), and that you have "driven" him or her to the problematic sexual behavior. When a sex addict is in the midst of active addiction, he or she may say cruel and heartless things.

Sometimes addiction first comes to light after the birth of a child. When some mothers are giving themselves to the task of taking care of the new addition to their family, they discover that their husband is acting out sexually. At this time of increased emotional vulnerability, her needs for appreciation, affection, and loyalty are met with rejection and abandonment.

For some women, the discovery of their partner's acting out may come as they have aged and their body has shown some of the natural effects of aging. If you are a woman to whom this has happened, you might have said to yourself, "Maybe it is my fault that my partner is acting out with other people." Regardless of what may have happened in your life or what your partner may have said to you, *his addiction is not your fault.*

As I noted earlier, some well-meaning therapists have wrongly advised women to buy sexy lingerie or to have sex with their partner more frequently as a way of "keeping him at home." This suggestion does not solve the problem of sex addiction but may actually feed it. Healthy sexuality dictates that people are only sexual when they feel like being sexual. A woman should not feel under any obligation to be sexual at times or in situations where she does not feel valued, loved, or safe.

This is true for men as well. As your partner's addiction has come to light, you may have tried in various ways to make yourself more attractive to him or her. And you may doubt yourself because your efforts to stimulate his or her interest in being sexual with you have been rebuffed. Perhaps your partner has even laughed at you or otherwise been cruel to you.

Especially in cases where the addiction is being fueled by pornography and masturbation, a natural consequence is for him or her to have less desire to be sexual with you. Your earnest attempts to impact the addiction by being sexier are likely to result in your feeling rejected, cheap, and foolish—they will not deflect the destructive behavior. The addiction concerns the addict directly; it is his or her responsibility. You did not cause the addiction. But you can be part of the solution by taking care of yourself, setting and enforcing healthy boundaries as to what is acceptable and what is unacceptable in your relationship, and doing your own recovery work, all the while encouraging your partner to embrace recovery.

Why Would Sex Addicts Return to Acting-Out Behavior When They Know That Such Behavior Is Damaging, Possibly Destroying Their Marriage or Intimate Relationship?

You caught her or him again! And once again, your partner promised that the addictive acting out would stop. Your spouse seems no less sincere than the first time he or she was caught. It just does not seem to add up.

The only adequate explanation as to why people continue such behavior in the face of such negative consequences is that they are caught in the grip of an active addiction that is characterized by obsessive thoughts, compulsive behaviors, and self-centered attitudes. For many people, both addicts and partners, the term *sex addiction* finally explains why a person would return to such incomprehensible and demoralizing behavior, as the AA Big Book says. Sane people would never risk their health, their relationship, their job, or, literally in some cases, their freedom for something as transient as sexual arousal. Yet we must assume that the 3 to 5 percent of all Americans who are sex addicts are not thinking clearly due to the changes in brain biochemistry that occur in addiction. Isn't that insanity? One can see how a doctor having too many drinks at a party risks his life, those of other drivers on the road, and his entire network of family, friends, and patients by thinking he can make it home on automatic pilot. It is that same form of insane thinking that leads the sex addict to believe his or her actions are under control and are no one else's business.

Addiction is about indulging in some of the most insane behavior in an effort to acquire the next fix, regardless of whether that fix comes from a substance or an activity. Nothing and no one matters to an active addict except that next high. Sex addiction is marked by brain changes and insane behavior, but sex addicts themselves remain solely responsible for their actions and for their recovery. No one made them pursue their sexual activity. Recovery is impossible until sex addicts face and own their behavior, without blaming anyone else, and determine that they are going to be accountable for their actions.

Is Sex Addiction Compulsive or Impulsive?

The answer is both. Sex addiction includes impulsive as well as compulsive behaviors. Certainly there is a compulsive element to sex addiction. Behaviors are repeated over and over again as sex addicts look for the high they received from their past acting out. Rituals often accompany the acting out so that addicts may wear the same clothes (or "lucky" underwear), cruise the same parts of town, spend hours surfing the Internet, or engage in other behaviors that are so regimented that it is almost as though the sex addict is following a script written by someone else. As one women said, "I was unable to stop using the Internet until the sun came up," or as one man reported, "When I finished with one prostitute I would immediately begin seeking the next."

There is also an impulsive element involved in sex addiction. For most sex addicts, there are times when they find their impulse to act out is triggered by something, then engage in sexual behavior they had not planned. Triggers may include seeing a provocative advertisement, passing a sex-oriented business, getting a phone call or email from a former acting-out partner, or opening an email only to find pornography. And without a good Personal Recovery Plan, proficiency in using the tools of recovery, and experience in keeping healthy boundaries, many such individuals find it difficult to resist the impulse to act out. Chapter 7 provides detailed information on developing a Personal Recovery Plan. Willpower alone is not enough to overcome a pattern of addictive behavior.

Many people struggling with sex addiction do not intend to act out. In fact, they may have made promises or vows (including to themselves) that they will never act out again. But then something associated with their sexual acting out triggers the impulse and they succumb to the same destructive behavior they swore they would never repeat. For the sex addict, as for all addicts, activation of the addiction itself is always within reach—unless one does the work of recovery and learns the skills of pushing back against the thoughts and impulses to act out through any of the manifestations of addiction, be it sex, substances, eating, or gambling.

If My Partner Is a Sex Addict, Is There Any Hope for My Relationship?

The answer is a qualified yes. The bad news is that sex addiction is one of the toughest addictions to conquer. (I use that word cautiously because it is never truly conquered, but it can be kept at bay for life.) Crack cocaine addiction is often thought to be among the most difficult forms of addiction to address, but clients I have treated who are addicted to both crack and sex tell me that recovery from their addiction to crack came more easily than recovery from their addiction to sex. Of course, recovery from addiction to sex is complicated by the fact that sex is a natural and healthy human drive. Total abstinence is possible and necessary in recovery from addiction to substances, whereas recovery from sex addiction involves reestablishing a healthy relationship to sex and keeping it in the context of a committed partnership, not giving it up permanently.

The good news is that sex addiction responds well to treatment. While I believe treatment by a competent sex addiction specialist is of paramount importance in recovery, some sex addicts never receive any kind of therapy or treatment and are able to achieve and maintain recovery through twelve-step fellowships. These groups, patterned after Alcoholics Anonymous (AA), go by names such as Sex Addicts Anonymous (SAA), Sexaholics Anonymous (SA), and Sex and Love Addicts Anonymous (SLAA). (A comprehensive listing of the twelve-step programs dedicated to helping sex addicts and their partners can be found in Appendix B.) The biggest determining factor in a person's success in recovery is his or her willingness to "go to any lengths," as it is described in twelve-step recovery, to get free from problematic sexual behavior.

For your relationship to survive after you enter recovery, there has to be a willingness from both your partner and you to do whatever it takes to make the relationship work. That will entail a lot of hard work for each of you. And it will require a willingness to stick with the relationship even when your friends or family members encourage you to leave. As long as your partner is actively pursuing recovery and you are working on your own recovery in therapy and through organizations like Co-Dependents of Sex Addicts (COSA), S-Anon, or Infidelity Survivors Anonymous (ISA) (see Appendix B), there is reason to believe that your relationship cannot only survive addiction, but actually thrive in recovery.

While there is no guarantee that your relationship will work, my experiences as a psychotherapist have shown that when both partners are committed to the relationship and are actively pursuing recovery with therapists trained to work with individuals where problematic sexual behavior is a factor, many of those relationships do indeed survive and thrive. Frequently, couples who are entering their second or third year of recovery state that their marriage/relationship is not only better than it was prior to the revelation of the addiction, but is actually better than they ever dreamed it could be.

Is Addiction a Choice?

This is a straightforward question that does not have a simple answer. There is certainly choice involved in a sex addict's behavior. Each person is responsible for the choices he or she makes and the consequences of his or her actions. But addiction is a powerful drive that creates changes in the brain chemistry of the addict, and these neurochemical alterations have direct and significant influences on behavior.

I have known men and women who are aware of the risks involved in their acting-out behavior but continue anyway. There are those who have been fired from multiple jobs for accessing pornography at work. I have known men who have repeatedly contracted sexually transmitted diseases and put their health and that of their partners at risk by habitually engaging in high-risk sexual behavior. Frequently, I talk to sex addicts who have destroyed multiple relationships and marriages due to their acting out. Why would a person return to risky behaviors in the face of such loss and pain?

The only thing that adequately explains such insane behavior in otherwise mentally competent individuals is addiction. No one chooses to become addicted—to anything. The process that leads to addiction begins with the choices a person makes. But with time and experience repeating the same destructive behaviors over and over, the obsessive thinking and compulsive behavior take on a life of their own and become less a matter of fully conscious choice and more of something the addict is driven toward. Sex addiction is more powerful than many people imagine. It is like an undertow that is always waiting to drag the individual under and carry him or her away.

Could My Partner Be Gay or Lesbian?

Sonny's Story

Sonny had been happily married for fifteen years. His wife had twice caught him in affairs and had been devastated by the knowledge that he had been emotionally involved with other women. Sonny did not want to hurt his wife anymore but did not feel he could completely stop acting out. He erroneously reasoned that the greatest problem was not that he was having sex outside their marriage but that he was involved with other women. Sonny thought that he could get some of the same sexual fulfillment with men. When he traveled on business, he sought sex with men by posting ads on various websites that had a "personals" section. Sonny believed himself to be heterosexual and even noted that when he would have sex with a man, the only way he could climax was to watch heterosexual pornography at the same time.

Upon finding out their partner has been having sex with men, often the first question women ask is, "Is my partner gay?" Certainly some men who act out with men are gay. However, there are a number of heterosexual men who act out with other men. Sonny is one of them. His acting out with men is something that he did for convenience and from a belief that it was not as great a betrayal to his wife. He just wanted to have sex, and he found an abundance of willing male partners who did not want a relationship but were also seeking sexual release.

This is a complicated issue. In terms of men acting out with other men, some women feel a bit of relief knowing their husband's acting out is not with women, while other women experience an extra measure of pain. For women who feel relieved, they may reason that their husband's behavior is not as much of a personal affront to them since their husband didn't look for sex with another woman. But for a number of women, the same-sex acting out of their husband brings additional questions, confusion, and perhaps shame.

There are numerous reasons that men might have sex with other men. Certainly one of the reasons is that the man identifies himself as gay. If this is the case and he chooses to live as a gay man, then each member of the family would benefit from some significant support (perhaps including psychotherapy for each person) as the man in question walks a new path and the rest of the family copes with his decision.

The purpose of this section is not to determine if a man is heterosexual, homosexual, or bisexual. There are numerous books devoted to this subject. Rather, this section asks you to consider the possibility that same-sex acting out is not the touchstone criterion to determine sexual orientation.

But If Your Male Partner Is Heterosexual, How Do You Explain the Fact That He Has Been Sexual with Other Men?

One of the reasons a heterosexual man may have sex with other men is to reenact past trauma that he experienced. If your husband was abused by a man or by a boy older than himself, he experienced some trauma as the result. One response to trauma is to unconsciously repeat the traumatizing event or events. Often these men are not conscious that they are reenacting their past traumatic experience. They do not have feelings of attraction for other men or yearn to have an emotional connection with them. All they know is that they have a desire to be sexual with men. As with all victims of abuse and trauma, these men should seek psychotherapy to cope with that past trauma.

Another reason heterosexual men may have sex with other men is that they are seeking a greater thrill because they consider this activity forbidden. The more forbidden, the greater the risk, and the greater the neurochemical reinforcement. Rather than being repelled by behavior they consider perverted, they become attracted to that which they once loathed.

Some men have sex with other men because they are seeking some sexual behavior they either do not experience with their partner or believe they would be criticized for seeking from their partner. Again, part of the thrill is crossing into the forbidden zone of sexual behaviors. They are able to get their sexual wants met without having to risk being rejected or ridiculed by their partner.

Still another reason heterosexual men may have sex with other men is that they may find a greater availability of partners—or at least they perceive that to be so. Public restrooms and parks have long been the hunting ground for men who are looking for male sex partners. The Internet brings multitudes of people willing to have anonymous sexual encounters into a public space. When some heterosexual men realize this, they become aware that sexual encounters are often available with little or no planning and may occupy only a few minutes of their time.

Heterosexual men may have anonymous sex with men because they feel the lack of emotional attachment makes those relationships safer. When they have sex with other men they rationalize that it is not cheating in the same sense it would be if they were having sex with a woman. They may tell themselves that they are still being faithful to their wives because they are not involved in a relationship that involves love or any emotional attachment.

When homosexual acting out occurs in a heterosexual relationship, in the majority of cases it concerns the male partner. As a generalization, men can cross over into homosexual activity and return to their heterosexual identity more easily than women can. The difference is one of emotional commitment and duration. Men typically do not need to make the same commitment of time and attention developing a relationship that a woman requires.

Traditionally, if a woman goes outside the primary relationship it is not to seek sexual pleasure per se, but emotional contact and communication. In terms of what men and women need in a relationship, a sense of dialogue, trust, and understanding are usually more necessary to women than to men. Usually, emotional intimacy precedes physical intimacy for women, whereas for men the emotional intimacy needn't be present. However, more women are creating alternate lives on the Internet, with women as well as men.

These conditions may change in our society as more and more people submerge their actual lives in virtual reality and create alternate identities through Internet interaction. It is difficult enough for a number of people to maintain a sense of integrity and selfhood in a world where deception, deceit, and illusion attempt to distract with sophisticated advertising, offering everything from a better vacation spot to the latest computer or tablet device. For the addict, though, the noise of temptation can be deafening.

Your Trauma

Lucy's Story

Lucy found out about her partner's clandestine sexual behavior six years ago. She confronted him and he told her it was all in her head. He convinced her that she was going crazy and that there was nothing going on. Anytime that she would mention to him that there were things about his behavior that did not make sense, her partner would yell at her and tell her she was stupid and insecure.

Two months ago, she confronted him with additional evidence that this time he did not even try to deny. He said he was relieved that he had been caught and that he was going to do all that he could to get free from that destructive behavior forever. And as far as Lucy knows, her partner is doing a good job with his recovery. However, Lucy's problems were just beginning. Sleep comes slowly for her now, and when it does come, it is frequently fitful. She awakens with nightmares involving her partner's sexual behavior. Some days she cannot eat. On other days Lucy is ravenous and devours any food in sight. She finds that staying busy helps, so she fills her days with activities and tries to think positive thoughts. But in unguarded moments Lucy breaks down in tears for no apparent reason. At other times she is gripped by fear but usually cannot pinpoint an event that has made her fearful. And at other times she rages at those closest to her.

Lucy finally saw a therapist who was well acquainted with sex addiction and with the impact of sexual addiction on partners. The therapist explained to Lucy that she was suffering from deep psychological trauma and suggested that she might have post-traumatic stress disorder, or PTSD. Lucy protested that this could not be the case since she had never served in the military and had not survived some type of catastrophe. Yet, as her therapist shared with her, there is a significant amount of evidence that some people who are in a relationship with someone who acts out sexually in ways that betray trust and shatter feelings of emotional safety can be traumatized and develop all of the symptoms of PTSD. For those partners who do not have PTSD, the effects of significant psychological trauma frequently still need to be addressed for them to heal.

Am I a "Co-addict"?

In the past much of the focus for the partners of sex addicts has been on recognizing and stopping codependent behaviors. To drive this point home, in some circles the partners of sex addicts have been considered "co-addicts." The intent was to help partners recognize that they have been part of the addicted-couple system, and therefore part of the problem, and that as such, they have their own healing work to do. I strongly disagree with the term *co-addict*. No one needs to be labeled or pathologized simply because they are in a relationship with a sex addict. In fact, that label is just another dimension of the trauma that some partners of sex addicts have to face. It may deepen guilt that they already feel if they see themselves as somehow responsible for their partner's sex addiction.

Similar terms are not used in any other chronic condition. For example, if a person develops type 2 diabetes, we understand that his or her condition is most likely due to genetic and lifestyle issues. The person's choices related to diet and lack of exercise have at the very least contributed to the disease. However, we would never call such a person's partner a "co-diabetic," even if that person prepared meals with a high fat content. We would say that the diabetic was responsible for what he or she ate.

Partners of sex addicts do have work to do. But the focus of their work early in recovery needs to be on self-care and trauma resolution. More attention is given to the subject of trauma in Chapter 12. As work continues, the focus expands to include identifying and modifying codependent behaviors that may be present, but in early recovery the focus should be on the trauma the partner suffers due to the behaviors of the sex addict.

CHAPTER 6

ADDRESSED TO THE COUPLE

In this chapter, I will use "you" to mean both the addict and the addict's partner, for in a relationship you are as one, and it is that unified force of love, spirit, and trust that must be brought back to health through recovery. Recovery means simultaneous hope for both of you. It means hope that your marriage or intimate relationship will not come to an end and that it can be restored.

Regardless of how bad things are in your relationship at present, regardless of how much trust you have lost, there is hope for you. Even if you cannot fully embrace this hope now, trust me when I say that after helping sex addicts free themselves and their loved ones from the grips of addiction, I have convincing proof that life can be different.

If you engage in recovery without reservation, it is possible to regain the relationship you lost, the relationship you thought was no longer possible to revive.

Is there really any freedom to be had on the recovery road? I wouldn't have devoted a significant portion of my life to helping sex addicts and their loved ones regain love and respect—their very lives—unless I believed totally in freedom from addiction. More specifically for you, I would not have written this book unless I knew this to be possible and wanted to share it with sex addicts and their partners everywhere. No matter where you are reading this, no matter how dark the place is where sex addiction has taken you, I want you to know that freedom is ahead if you both commit yourselves to recovery.

The addict has a much harder road to take if he or she must take it alone. The emotional and physical presence of a partner adds comfort and strength during the process. I have observed a great truth: When the sex addict embraces recovery, when it becomes an all-consuming passion, he or she will achieve freedom from problematic sexual behaviors. Within a relatively short time the individual suffering from addiction will find that life can be free of acting out. This may come almost as the fulfillment of a dream. Prior to recovery, a number of sex addicts believe they will never get free from the demoralizing and often dangerous behaviors that have defined their lives. Some are reconciled to the belief that they are not capable of being monogamous. Others are resigned to the belief that their addiction will eventually put an end to everything that is of value to them.

Addiction is generally considered, including by most experts, to be an incurable condition that will continue to follow a person throughout life. That does not mean that sex addicts in recovery will struggle daily with whether or not they will act out. Sex addiction can be managed effectively through the process of recovery. This requires recovering addicts to remain forever vigilant to the insidious and surreptitious nature of addiction to keep from returning to their destructive behaviors.

Recovering sex addicts must realize that they can never take their behavior for granted. While focusing on maintaining their recovery one day at a time, there will be places they will never again be able to visit; they will always need to avoid certain kinds of movies and television shows, and they will likely even have to forgo listening to certain songs or perhaps whole categories of music because it was once closely tied to their acting out.

These boundaries are not imposed by a partner or a therapist or a twelve-step sponsor. Instead, when sex addicts have gotten fully into recovery and begin to understand what is required for the recovery journey, they impose boundaries on themselves. This enables them to live with what has been described by sex addicts themselves as a "caged tiger."

The freedom that you both will ultimately experience is freedom from fear. The addict will no longer feel that he or she has to lie or be deceitful. The partner will no longer have to question the truthfulness of what the recovering addict tells him or her, even regarding areas that have caused conflict and pain in the past. The recovery journey requires that an addict learn to live in the truth. This may ultimately prove to be more difficult than the ability to stop acting out. In active addiction, lying and deception become intertwined with daily life. But recovery will ultimately bring freedom from deception as the sex addict learns to speak the truth in all areas of life. If the addict becomes fully engaged in recovery and is willing to do whatever it takes to get "sexually sober" and stay that way, you will find that the fear of acting out will diminish.

CHAPTER 7

RECOVERY COMPONENTS

Recovery Timetable

How long will recovery last? There are two answers. The first answer is that recovery is a lifelong process that never ends. Sex addicts never get to a place where they can declare they have been cured and are fully "recovered." Early recovery is the most challenging part of the process. After approximately three to five years, one's recovery achieves a stability that decreases the risk of relapse into sexual acting out. However, the person will always be "in recovery," and must remain vigilant because no one is ever exempt from the possibility of relapse.

Factors Affecting Treatment and Recovery

There are numerous factors that affect the course of recovery from sex addiction. The crisis that brought about the initial search for recovery must be great enough to motivate the sex addict to be willing to look for outside help. It is not enough that life has become difficult or that there is discord in the relationship. It typically takes a significant crisis to propel a sex addict to take the plunge into recovery. The early months are often significantly impacted by the presence of the dual enemies of recovery—denial and resistance.[15]

DENIAL

Denial is a defense mechanism that sex addicts use in order to be able to live with themselves in spite of the presence of behaviors that they often abhor. To keep from being plunged into the depths of despair, sex addicts may become skilled at denying not only that they are addicted to sex, but that there is anything wrong with their behavior. They can find numerous examples in society and especially in entertainment that validate their belief that they are normal and just doing what other people are doing. This denial is so strong that some sex addicts can live in this state for years without giving much thought to wanting to stop their compulsive behavior. Tragically, some are never able to break free from denial. They live with the belief that their behaviors are typical of others and they ignore all evidence to the contrary.

RESISTANCE

Resistance is a defense mechanism firmly entrenched in sex addicts who resist all efforts by their partner, their family, and their friends to get them into recovery. In therapy, resistance results in slow progress or no progress at all. It is characteristic of a client who is resistant to treatment to challenge therapeutic interventions and assignments. Clients who are highly resistant believe they have great insight into their addiction and that they know best what treatment they need. They may even go from therapist to therapist as they shop for someone who will agree with the treatment philosophy and approach they demand.

There are a number of reasons that addicts have resistance. The most common is that they may view the term *sex addict* as so negative that they will avoid identifying themselves with it at all costs. Others resist treatment because they do not believe anyone else is like them and therefore they do not fit into treatment plans that are designed for sex addicts. Some individuals are resistant because they are fearful they will have to give up sex for life, and they do not believe that will be possible.

Resistance and denial present challenges in treatment. Only when sex addicts are able to break through both of these defense mechanisms are they able to make significant progress in treatment and recovery. Some sex addicts continue to exhibit resistance and denial for years, resulting in little change in their behavior and great frustration for their partners.

Partner Participation in Recovery

Another significant factor in determining the course of recovery is the partner's willingness to participate. Unfortunately, there are partners who refuse to do any work in recovery. They reason that since the addiction pertains to their partner, it is up to him or her to get fixed. Sadly, such partners fail to see that their own pain and trauma are being prolonged when they refuse to participate in the addict's recovery as well as in the process of recovery for themselves. Importantly, they are also choosing to ignore the fact that it will take the work of both partners to rebuild the marriage or relationship.

From a relationship standpoint, both partners need to be willing to do the work of their individual recovery first, and then focus on working on the relationship if there is to be any hope of restoring it. The relationship may be the first thing a couple wants to see restored. However, individual recovery is foundational to couples recovery. Recovery progresses through readily identifiable phases. With each phase the sex addict and partner move toward the goal of completely arresting the addiction and restoring their relationship.

As this process proceeds, the sex addict and the partner will be able to determine if solid recovery is taking place by checking their progress against the Hallmarks of Good Recovery (discussed later in this chapter). In the process, my approach calls for both to produce a Personal Recovery Plan as a guide for their recovery.

Recovery Phases

Survival Phase	This phase starts when recovery begins and lasts from 6 months to 1 year or more.
Stability Phase	Begins from 6 months to 2 years into recovery and lasts 1 year or more.
Sustaining Phase	Begins from 1½ to 3 years into recovery and lasts 1 year or more.
Freedom Phase	Persons in this phase have been in recovery for 2½ years or more. This is the ultimate phase one aspires to reach in recovery.

SURVIVAL PHASE

This is the beginning of the recovery journey. The survival phase lasts from six months to a year or more. This phase does not begin until a person recognizes he or she is a sex addict and is willing to get help. He or she may still have significant denial and resistance in place and may not know a lot about what is required, but at least he or she has started the journey. The focus of therapy in this phase of recovery is on stopping all acting-out behaviors. It is during this phase that sex addicts must break through both denial and resistance. Success in recovery depends on effectively dealing with both of these defense mechanisms.

A common denominator in this phase is the crisis that led to the addict's admission that his or her life has become unmanageable to the point where he or she is open to the need to change. The crises in the addict's relationship, on the job, or in the legal system have finally gotten his or her attention, and he or she is desperate for help. However, if the crisis is viewed as temporary or just an inconvenience to be weathered before returning to previous patterns, sex addicts may wander in and out of this phase over a period of years before actually making a commitment to recovery.

In the survival phase sex addicts first attend twelve-step meetings and may seek out a therapist concerning their addiction. Group therapy is often started a few months into recovery as an adjunct to individual therapy, and provides important opportunities for mutual support and identification. Some individuals believe life as they know it ends at this point. And perhaps it does. If all they have known is sex addiction and out-of-control problematic sexual behavior, then if they maintain their recovery, that life of acting out is coming to an end.

While this is usually the beginning of the recovery journey, persons who have suffered a slip or relapse are also in the survival phase. While a slip or a relapse does not mean a person loses what he or she has learned in recovery thus far, it does mean that there is more work to do that necessitates a return to those basic principles of recovery in order to set the stage for further progress.

Persons who have been in recovery for some time but are currently experiencing a crisis related to the consequences of their addictive behavior that is now affecting them are also in the survival phase.

Not only does therapy in this phase focus on stopping all problematic sexual behaviors, it also lays the foundation for future recovery work. This is a time for establishing solid sexual sobriety and being able to identify, on a calendar, a sobriety date. During this phase, all immediate crises are addressed, and a preliminary plan for recovery is mapped out. By *sobriety* I am referring to the total absence of behaviors that a sex addict has defined for him- or herself as being "forbidden." For example, in a marriage or committed relationship, that usually includes being sexual with anyone other than one's partner. Sobriety can be lost or broken. In contrast, the process of recovery can continue even if there is a setback in the form of a slip or relapse.

Couples therapy in this phase is specific to crisis management and facilitating an understanding of the role that each partner plays in the recovery process, and how the individual recovery of each partner is crucial for the relationship to succeed. There is also a focus on laying a foundation upon which trust can be built in the future. It may be a while before any real trust is built, but at least there can be work in this area that down the road can help in the restoration of trust.

As a recovering sex addict moves out of this phase, he or she will have firmly established sobriety as it relates to inappropriate sexual activity. All problematic sexual behaviors will have ended. The individual will be engaged in regular recovery routines apart from therapy, including consistently attending twelve-step meetings and working with a sponsor.

STABILITY PHASE
This phase begins six months to two years into recovery and lasts for a year or more. Persons in this recovery phase have a good understanding of recovery and are regularly engaged in the recovery basics. They continue to attend twelve-step meetings regularly and work actively with their sponsor as they progress through the steps as outlined by the twelve-step fellowship with which they are affiliated.

The focus of therapy in this phase is on making recovery routines consistent habits and accepting that recovery is a lifelong process. Clients typically have let go of their denial and resistance and are making solid progress in recovery. They look forward to attending twelve-step meetings and recognize therapy as something that enhances their recovery rather than as a punishment for previous bad behavior. Another significant focus of therapy in this phase is on relapse prevention. Starting a process of recovery is not difficult, but staying in recovery is. With this in mind, therapists help equip clients with tools for dealing with triggers that activate urges to act out. This phase further prepares clients for various recovery challenges and for taking greater responsibility for their own recovery.

It is during this phase that traditional couples therapy can begin. Communication techniques are taught, and couples learn basic dialogue skills that allow them to communicate with each other without blaming and shaming. Conflict resolution is also taught and practiced during this phase.

Several significant things have happened in recovery as a client moves to the next phase. First, he or she will have made a complete disclosure of all of his or her acting-out behavior to his or her partner. The client has taken and passed a polygraph exam to verify that the disclosure is accurate and complete. (It should be noted that a number of clients complete this during the survival recovery phase.) Next, the client will be living "slip-free" and have been free from all acting-out behaviors for at least six months. At this point sex addicts do not see the responsibility for using tools of recovery as a burden but as a means of achieving freedom from their compulsive behaviors and restoring integrity. Partners moving out of this phase are actively working on their own recovery, and the relationship has been stabilized around recovery norms. Recovery has, in effect, become the couple's new normal.

Before moving toward a polygraph exam, read the next three chapters. Polygraph can be a helpful tool in recovery *when* it is part of an integrated therapeutic approach. Used by itself, polygraph is not necessarily helpful to recovery and may indeed be harmful. A complete discussion of the appropriate use of polygraph exams is found in Chapter 9.

SUSTAINING PHASE

This phase begins eighteen months to three years into recovery and lasts for one year or more. Clients at this phase have assumed total responsibility for their own recovery. Disclosure has been accomplished, and the relationship has been stabilized. Sexual sobriety is solid and growing. The focus on therapy during this phase of recovery is on deepening the addict's knowledge and broadening the foundation of recovery. Therapy may move from a weekly to a biweekly routine. Couples therapy during this phase is focused on understanding and developing healthy sexuality. This is an often-overlooked subject in recovery but one that demands significant attention. It is not enough that all problematic sexual behaviors be stopped; couples need to learn how to relate sexually in a healthy manner.

As a client moves out of this stage of recovery, he or she has worked all of the steps of recovery in one of the twelve-step fellowships. The recovering sex addict will be free from all acting-out behaviors for a minimum of one year. By this time, his or her anger and resentment are well managed, and the relationship with his or her partner is growing as both trust and intimacy are being rebuilt.

FREEDOM PHASE

Persons in this phase have been in recovery for two and a half years or more. They typically spend the first six to twelve months in this phase actively working on recovery. Clients in this phase ultimately move out of therapy or use therapy sporadically to address specific concerns, work on rough spots in their relationships, or do periodic recovery checkups. The focus of therapy during this phase is to fine-tune recovery routines. Tools and recovery techniques that were learned early in recovery are reviewed. There is an emphasis on establishing balance in the client's life.

Work with couples in this stage is focused on deepening and expanding skills learned earlier. Communication and conflict-resolution techniques are reviewed. There is a significant emphasis on boundaries as well as continued work in the area of healthy sexuality. As clients move out of therapy, they will have been free from all acting-out behaviors for at least two years. By this time they are actively sponsoring others in their twelve-step program and are otherwise engaged in giving back to the recovery community. They have developed and implemented a strong maintenance plan for continued recovery. The time comes for therapy to end when the couple's relationship is stable and growing. The relationship is not without conflict, but the couple has learned to resolve conflicts without attacking or shaming each other. Trust has been substantially and perhaps completely restored in the relationship. With measured steps, hope has led to freedom.

Recovery Timeline

PHASES OF RECOVERY TIMELINE

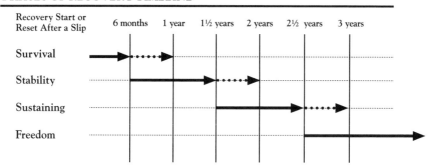

Recovery Is Something a Person Does!

The word *recovery* can be used in many ways as it pertains to sex addiction. Recovery can describe the goal of a person and also his or her state of mind. Recovery can be used to describe the journey one takes in getting his or her life back. Ultimately, recovery is a state of both mind and being, and a set of actions. While individuals say they are "in recovery," unless they are taking recovery-related action to back up that self-identification, they are at risk of returning to their problematic sexual behavior and active addiction. What does quality recovery look like? Persons who are in recovery are engaged in doing the work of recovery. When a person is in recovery, there is ample evidence of involvement in recovery activities.

Hallmarks of Quality Recovery

At the beginning of therapy, I provide clients with an understanding of sex addiction and also give them an overview of recovery. In the first or second therapy session, I lay out the various action items that are involved in recovery. There are things to be done immediately, as well as things the recovering sex addict will need to do daily, weekly, monthly, and annually.

Start attending twelve-step meetings. From the first day of recovery it is essential to take significant steps to address the addiction. The first thing the sex addict must do is find a list of twelve-step groups that support sex addiction recovery in his or her area. You can find a list of these groups in Appendix B. Attend a minimum of two twelve-step meetings a week. Many recovering addicts find attending ninety meetings in ninety days (a "90/90") an effective way to build a foundation for recovery.

Get a sponsor. Sponsors are recovering addicts with experience in the twelve-step program, who know the Twelve Steps and have worked them with a sponsor themselves, and have a significant period of time—ideally a year or more—in sexual sobriety. A sponsor's role is to provide a source of support and accountability. A sponsor provides further accountability for the sex addict and serves as a mentor in recovery, guiding him or her through the Twelve Steps. Regular contact with a sponsor is an important part of one's ongoing recovery routine.

When a person first reads the Twelve Steps, it may not be apparent that working these steps involves a significant amount of work. While there is not one right way to work the steps, each sponsor has his or her own approach to methodically guide sex addicts through this experiential process of growth and healing over a period of several months to a year or more. After completing this work with a sponsor and maintaining sexual sobriety, the recovering addict is then qualified to become a sponsor and guide other recovering persons through the steps of recovery.

Circle of Five. The addict is encouraged to establish a Circle of Five—a group of five people of the same gender to whom he or she will continually be accountable. The members of this circle know all about his or her addiction and will be open to regular contact with him or her. Typically, these will be other persons in recovery from sex addiction whom the individual can immediately contact if necessary.

A Circle of Five is particularly important for men since they have a tendency to isolate themselves and to try to handle problems on their own, whereas women are more relational and are more comfortable sharing their feelings with other women. This reluctance to be open is why some men refuse to ask for directions or ask a neighbor for help moving a heavy object. Men are often acculturated to believe they need to handle things by themselves and that it may even be a sign of weakness to ask for help. When a man is struggling with problematic sexual behavior, he may become more isolated. He may stop having contact with friends. He may even cut himself off from family members when his acting out is at its peak.

With a sponsor and a Circle of Five, the recovering addict will always have access to a personal support system that goes beyond just attending twelve-step meetings.

Begin therapy with a sex addiction therapist. Is it mandatory that a sex addict engage the services of a psychotherapist for recovery? The short answer is no. A significant portion of sex addicts do not use the services of a therapist. And for persons who simply cannot afford therapy, they can establish solid recovery by utilizing twelve-step groups and maintaining a regular working relationship with their sponsor.

But it is also true that many sex addicts struggle to establish and maintain recovery without professional assistance. Often therapists are able to help recovering persons develop a better recovery foundation than they could otherwise. If you choose to use a therapist, be sure you select a therapist who is skilled in working with persons who struggle with problematic sexual behavior. Good places to begin this search are the Society for the Advancement of Sexual Health (www.sash.net) and the International Institute for Trauma and Addiction Professionals (www.iitap.com). In my professional experience, therapy with a sex addiction therapist should begin immediately and should continue for two to three years. A combination of individual and group therapy creates an effective way of treating sexual addiction.

Personal Recovery Plan

While there are many elements to recovery and no two recovery plans are exactly the same, each person in recovery must come up with his or her own Personal Recovery Plan in consultation with his or her therapist or, in the absence of a sex addiction therapist, his or her sponsor. Each plan will include a list of actions a person is to take on a daily, weekly, monthly, and annual basis. After clients have put together a first draft of their Personal Recovery Plan, they are guided through the following checklist to see if there are additional elements that need to be added.

Recovery is most successful when multiple routines are built into regular daily and weekly activities. The more structure there is, the more effective the recovery plan becomes. Routine and structure assist successful recovery. Both the sex addict and the partner should develop their own Personal Recovery Plans. The following material covers numerous items that are essential to a Personal Recovery Plan. Quite a few of them are specific to the sex addict, but some are also applicable to the partner.

PERSONAL RECOVERY PLAN: IMMEDIATELY

(Although these items were mentioned earlier, they are important enough to include again here.)

• Change cell phone number(s). The only exception is if this number has *never* been used in acting out and/or contacting acting-out partners.

- Change email address(es). The only exception is if this address has *never* been used in acting out and/or contacting acting-out partners.

- Close all "extra" or secret email accounts.

- Close all secret bank and credit card accounts.

- Eliminate pornography stash. This step should be taken with the help of a sponsor or a trusted friend who is also in recovery. The additional accountability afforded by this person will lessen the possibility of retaining certain "favorite" items that have the potential to trigger a descent back into active addiction. Your goal is to lay a solid foundation for recovery.

- Make a commitment to *stay* in recovery *and do whatever it takes* to be free from acting out!

- See a psychiatrist. A significant number of sex addicts suffer from depression or other disorders that can make recovery difficult or impossible if not treated. If attention deficit hyperactivity disorder (ADHD) is present, it too must be diagnosed and treated in order for recovery to be successful.

- Attend an "S" twelve-step group meeting today. For twelve-step fellowships and meeting locations in your area, see Appendix B.

- Get a twelve-step program sponsor.

- Purchase and work through the workbook *Thirty Days to Hope & Freedom from Sexual Addiction: The Essential Guide to Beginning Recovery and Preventing Relapse*. Also get a copy of the "I Can Stop" video series that accompanies the workbook. Both are available at www.hopeandfreedom.com.

PERSONAL RECOVERY PLAN: DAILY

- Read the daily meditation from *Answers in the Heart*, found at the Recovery-Related Books link at www.hopeandfreedom.com. Whatever your spiritual beliefs, be sure to embrace the spiritual aspect of your life during recovery.

- Morning prayer for sexual sobriety and recovery. This can be basic and nondenominational, such as a simple request like "Thank you for a day of sobriety yesterday. Help me to live in recovery today."

- Do step work. Your sponsor will lead you in working the steps.

- Read the basic textbook of the "S" group you attend (sex addiction twelve-step fellowship) cover to cover, and read it over again. This text is published by each of the twelve-step groups that focus on problematic sexual behavior. In each book you will find information about the distinctive features of that group as well as practical recovery suggestions.

- Restrict or eliminate TV watching. A good exercise at the beginning of recovery is to make a log of your weekly use of time. Keep track of how much time you spend in each activity by quarter-hour increments. It may be surprising how much time is wasted in watching television and in nonproductive surfing of the Internet.

- Strictly limit computer use. Beyond what is required for your job, determine the maximum amount of time you will spend on computer entertainment pursuits daily. Set yourself this boundary and rigorously maintain it. Consider completely curtailing evening computer use.

- Avoid music and movies that do not support recovery. For some this may mean they have to eliminate a particular genre of music. For others there may be selected songs as well as movies that they choose to avoid in the interest of their recovery.

- Develop healthy eating habits.

- Limit or avoid caffeine.

- Limit or eliminate alcohol.

- No illegal drugs. Take prescription medications only as directed. Be advised that certain types of medications, including painkillers, anti-anxiety agents, and sleep aids can be highly addictive.

- Get regular sleep—a minimum of seven to eight hours a night.

- Journal. Make daily recovery-related journal entries that include your thoughts, your feelings, and the areas in which you are doing well and those where you may be struggling.

- Affirmations. Claim a new affirmation every morning and repeat that affirmation out loud at least 100 times during the day. In this way, you can replace negative thoughts and destructive self-talk with positive self-talk.

- Evening meditation or devotional. If married or in a committed relationship, try doing this with your partner.

- Evening prayer for sexual sobriety and continued recovery.

PERSONAL RECOVERY PLAN: WEEKLY

- Review journal entries for the past week. Do some weekly goal setting in your journal.

- Individual therapy session.

- Group therapy (usually after being in individual therapy for a few months).

- Attend a minimum of two twelve-step meetings. Many sex addicts find attending ninety meetings in ninety days ("90/90") a good way to establish recovery.

- Do some service work in twelve-step meetings. (This is simply finding a way of helping out, such as preparing the location for a meeting, cleaning up after a meeting, or providing another service for the twelve-step fellowship.)

- Meet face-to-face with your sponsor.

- Establish a Circle of Five.

- FASTT Check-In with partner (explained in detail in Chapter 16).

- Make a minimum of two "program calls" (phoning other persons in recovery to talk about recovery progress—this is also good practice in case you experience an emergency and need to reach out to others for assistance).

- Physical exercise—a minimum of three times a week for thirty minutes each time.

- Worship or some other weekly spiritual discipline. Don't neglect the spiritual dimension of your recovery.

- Do something fun for yourself.

- Date night with spouse or significant other.

PERSONAL RECOVERY PLAN: MONTHLY

- Review all journal entries for the past month.

- If not in regular weekly therapy, consider having a monthly session for guidance and as an additional point of accountability.

- Joint therapy session with partner (if in a committed relationship).

PERSONAL RECOVERY PLAN: ANNUALLY

- Marriage enrichment seminar/conference (if married).

- Weekend retreat for men only or women only: Attend at least one retreat (twelve-step, therapist-led, or spiritual) each year.

- Physical exam. Physical health is often neglected while living in addiction.

- Dental exams twice a year.

PERSONAL RECOVERY PLAN

Things I Commit to Doing for My Recovery

What I need to do with regard to recovery, physical health, and spiritual and mental well-being, and for my relationship.

DAILY	WEEKLY	MONTHLY
1. Morning prayer for recovery	1. Attend twelve-step meetings	1.
2.	2. Meet with my sponsor	2.
3.	3.	3.
4.	4.	4.
5.	5.	5.
6.	6.	6.
7.	7.	7.
8.	8.	8.
9.	9.	9.
10.	10.	10.
11.	11.	11.
12.	12.	12.
13.	13.	13.
14.	14.	14.
15. Evening prayer for recovery	15.	15.

ANNUAL ACTIVITIES/COMMITMENTS

1. Physical exam	3.	5.
2. Dental checkup (2 times)	4.	6.

You may find this list daunting. Remember, your addiction to sex is deeply ingrained and has become a way of life. It will take considerable effort to overcome your destructive habit patterns. If this seems like too much work, *perhaps you are not ready for recovery*. Hopefully, you and those you love will not have to suffer much more before you are ready to make recovery a way of life.

A Special Message to the Deeply Religious

There is a tendency after having a deeply moving religious or spiritual experience to believe that you no longer have a problem with sex addiction. People will announce they have been healed or delivered from their addiction. And on the surface this seems like a great experience to have.

The question is not "Is God able to heal?" but "Are you able to continue to live as God wants you to live?" Sex addiction is as real as a heart attack. Pray for healing. Then do those things that are necessary to stay in good health. Be careful of the hubris that comes from setting yourself up as someone who has been healed or delivered. Some believe that if they declare they have been delivered loud enough and long enough, their deliverance or healing will be accomplished. Often what is behind such declarations is a belief that the person making the declaration should be exempted from the hard work of recovery. Such persons believe they do not need to attend twelve-step meetings, get a sponsor, or work the steps like "ordinary" people.

A much more helpful path is to treasure any deeply moving spiritual experiences that you have. You can continue to believe you have been delivered or healed. But continue doing the work of recovery without making announcements, and focus on maintaining your spiritual standing. Then when you are ninety years of age, if you have been completely free from all acting out, you can declare to others that you have been healed.

Taking an example from Christianity. If ever there was someone who was so close to the Lord that he should be able to claim the spiritual elite status of being healed, it was the apostle Paul. Yet this stalwart saint declared, "I want to do what is right, but I can't. I want to do what is good, but I don't. I don't want to do what is wrong, but I do it anyway."[16]

When a client tells me he has been delivered from sex addiction, I also usually hear him saying that he does not have to attend twelve-step meetings, work the steps of recovery, use the tools of recovery, or do anything to remain sexually sober. What I find interesting is that many of these people have had other deeply moving spiritual experiences in the past where they declared themselves to be healed from sex addiction, only to fall back into their old behaviors after a brief period free from acting out.

If a sex addict wants to believe he or she has been healed or delivered from his or her addiction, I caution him or her to keep those thoughts personal rather than share them publicly, and continue the disciplines of recovery. God can change your heart. But you need to change your habits. Lean on your faith. Pray like it all depends on God. Then get off your knees and do the work of recovery like it all depends on you.

CHAPTER 8

DISCLOSURE

Daniel's Story

Disclosure may bring terror into the heart of both the sex addict and the partner. Daniel dreaded disclosure from the first time he heard someone mention it in his twelve-step group. While he did not mention it then to his partner, Teri, he was fearful that she also might hear about disclosure, and if she did, he was sure that she would insist that he do a full disclosure to her of all of his acting-out behavior. There were things, many things, that he had never told another soul. He was sure that if Teri knew what he had done since they had been together, she would leave him. Not only were there things he had never told her, but he purposely hid the magnitude of his acting out in the years before he met Teri.

He recalled when they were telling each other about their sexual history. He listened to Teri as she told him about her previous sexual encounters. Daniel sanitized his sexual history so that it would match Teri's and, in his mind, make him more acceptable to the woman with whom he wanted to share the rest of his life. When he finished, Teri remarked that she was surprised he had not been involved in more sexual behavior. He replied that he had been saving himself for her. But now he was fearful she would eventually find out the whole truth about his sexual behavior, and he was sure that would mark the end of the relationship.

There are relationships that end after disclosures. However, when a disclosure is done with the aid of a skilled sex addiction therapist, many relationships not only survive but can ultimately thrive after the acting out has ceased, significant recovery has been accomplished, and trust has been restored.

What Is Disclosure?

Disclosure in recovery is a clinical process of revealing all of one's past acting-out behaviors in the interest of ending secrets, getting honest, and restoring integrity. The purpose of a full disclosure is to clear the slate, put an end to acting out, and create an opportunity to rebuild the relationship.

What is disclosure? The *American Heritage Dictionary* defines disclosure as

1. The act or process of revealing or uncovering.

2. Something uncovered; a revelation.[17]

There are different types and levels of disclosure. As a sex addict begins working with a sponsor in a twelve-step program of recovery, it is critical for him or her to be open and honest with his or her sponsor about all behaviors. The disclosure that is the focus of this chapter is the truth-telling that a sex addict does with his or her partner during recovery. In this disclosure, the individual tells his or her partner every part of his or her sexual history, omitting nothing. As intimidating as this might seem, the goal is to get rid of all secrets and begin the process of washing away the shame that accompanies them. Believe it or not, as difficult as the process can be, it is very effective. As a clinical procedure, disclosures are carefully planned and require a significant amount of preparation. It is recommended that disclosure be conducted with the assistance of a skilled sex addiction therapist during a therapy session.

To many people, even the mention of the word *disclosure* brings a mix of fear and promise to both sex addicts and their partners. Disclosure is championed by some and denigrated by others. There is debate in twelve-step groups about the advisability of doing a disclosure. Some people in recovery advocate for it, while others believe it is harmful to recovery. They recount "people they know" who have done a disclosure that turned out badly. They may tell of their own experiences with disclosure and the damage they believe it did to a relationship. Some speak with passion about how the Ninth Step says amends are to be made only when they will not harm others. Some individuals believe that disclosure will harm their spouse and themselves if they reveal all of their acting-out behaviors.

Recovery is a program of rigorous honesty. How can one be honest and not tell the whole truth to his or her partner about his or her behavior during their relationship? The "Big Book" of Alcoholics Anonymous states that those who don't recover are people who are "constitutionally incapable of being honest."[18] Recovery requires honesty. Although disclosure is not part of twelve-step work and is not synonymous with the Ninth Step, it is an important element of recovery that is utilized in professionally facilitated therapy.

Disclosure, as used in sex addiction recovery, is not a way for the sex addict to unload all of his or her shame and guilt onto his or her partner. It is not a lengthy conversation in the bedroom where a partner describes all the lurid details of past sexual exploits and transgressions. This type of confession is damaging if the partner is not prepared to hear it, and does not have any psychological protection after the disclosure. To worsen the experience, this type of informational and emotional "dumping" is usually incomplete, inflicting further trauma on the partner when the sex addict later recalls additional details of acting out.

It can take time in recovery before the addict is ready to be completely truthful in disclosing the extent of his or her sexual acting out. Deception is so ingrained in sex addicts that it often takes a period of time before they are ready to be completely open and honest with the therapist, as well as with their partner. I hear of many incidents of acting out a year after a person starts therapy for sex addiction, when the person previously stated that he or she had told "everything." It sometimes takes even longer for sex addicts to get to the point where they are ready to be truthful with their partners.

Disclosure is a clinical procedure that takes place only after preparation of both the sex addict and the partner, and is guided by a well-trained sex addiction therapist as part of the treatment process. Disclosure needs to be conducted according to specific guidelines that will be covered in detail later in this chapter. Disclosures should be conducted only after the sex addict has stopped all acting out. If the addict is not ready to make a break with his or her past behavior, the disclosure will have to be repeated, further traumatizing the partner. This retraumatization is evident when addicts make partial or progressive disclosures. Some sex addicts prefer making a partial disclosure, usually in an attempt to minimize damage to the relationship. If, later on, they deem their partner strong enough, they may reveal additional information. In fact, partial disclosure is in many ways worse than no disclosure at all.

One research study found that multiple disclosures are common and damaging. Schneider, Corley, and Irons found a majority of sex addicts (58.7 percent) and partners (69.7 percent) reported that there had been more than one major disclosure. In some of the cases, the intent was for the first partial disclosure to be sufficient and to answer the questions of the partner.[19] But revelations of additional acting-out behavior or discovery of more secret sexual behavior prompts another disclosure.

Part of the preparation for disclosure is for the addict to carefully examine his or her past. It is helpful for recovering addicts to do a careful reconstruction of past sexual history prior to disclosure. When I review their sexual histories with clients, frequently they say that they had completely forgotten certain events until we started working together to uncover their past behaviors. The reason sex addicts have such difficulty with their memory is that they have spent years trying to forget, often subconsciously, what they had done. Denying past events and forgetting them is one way they cope with bad behaviors, but it is a poor one.

There are times when addicts make their disclosure to the wrong person. After reaching the point of recognizing their addictive behavior and how destructive it is, some addicts decide to "come clean" with their employers. They reveal that they have not been as productive as they could have been due to their addiction. In some cases, recovering addicts feel compelled to tell their employers they used company time or perhaps a company computer for acting out. As genuine as the motives may be to reveal this sexual behavior to one's employer, doing so often has negative consequences. One reason is that sexual addiction is not always well understood by employers and not covered by benefit plans or employee assistance programs, as is addiction to alcohol and other drugs. Unfortunately, the response of some employers upon learning an employee is acting out sexually is immediate termination.

Rather than making a disclosure to an employer that may be premature or inappropriate, I counsel clients to wait before approaching their employer about their problematic sexual behavior. If a disclosure is indicated, there is adequate time to do this in the future. I encourage clients to wait until the Eighth and Ninth Steps in their twelve-step work and let their sponsor help them explore the options for making amends to their employer. In some cases the amends may come in the form of an anonymous donation to a charity in the name of the employer. Or in cases involving theft, full financial restitution may be made anonymously.

Another well-intentioned but misguided disclosure is to disclose sexual acting out to casual friends. Recovering sex addicts may be so excited about their entry into recovery and their newfound freedom that they are tempted to blurt out indiscriminately that they are sex addicts in recovery. While one can praise their enthusiasm and wish to share their delight, the potential for such disclosures to turn out badly outweighs the temporary joy received from telling others about their recovery journey.

Another mistake is disclosing to children any details inappropriate for a child's age. This should be avoided. It is also not advisable to make a disclosure to children before making a disclosure to one's spouse. When making a disclosure to children, the parents should do so together.

Children need to have an opportunity to hear from the addict about the behavior and recovery rather than having the other parent disclose it. Disclosures must be age-appropriate, and disclosures to the children, even adult children, do not require the same level of detail as disclosures to the spouse. The disclosure should focus on the fact that the improper behavior has stopped and the parent is in recovery. Equally important is for the spouse of the addict to refrain from using shaming or blaming language in front of the children.

The process of disclosing the extent and depth of an addict's sexual acting out often follows a predictable course. First, there is complete denial by the addict. Even faced with irrefutable evidence, some addicts adamantly deny any wrongdoing. Some, faced with photos of their car in front of a strip club, deny that it is their vehicle. When it is pointed out that the car has their license number, they insist the photo was altered. There are female addicts who, having received expensive gifts from sex partners, concoct stories to attempt to explain the gifts and shield the sexual behavior. Anger often follows denial. The anger may take the form of self-righteous indignation: When confronted, the addict says, "I can't believe you would accuse me of such things!" Anger may be followed by a wall of silence.

Sensing he or she may no longer be able to get by with alibis, the sex addict may make a partial disclosure consisting of half-truths after being caught, followed by new alibis and additional partial disclosures of acting-out behavior. The final step in this journey is when a complete disclosure is made. A full disclosure can come only when the addict gets to the point where recovery and regaining integrity are more important than guarding secrets. When a sex addict gets to the point of committing to make a full and complete disclosure, he or she can make significant gains in recovery.

Disclosure, Hope & Freedom Style

The following is the procedure used by Hope & Freedom Counseling Services many times during disclosure.[20] Other sex addiction therapists' disclosure procedures may be different.

We have used disclosure in two ways. The major focus of our practice is working with couples in Three-Day Intensives, which are three days of concentrated work with couples that focuses on showing the addict how to become free from all addictive behaviors, supporting the partner in the trauma caused by the addict's acting out, showing the addict how to be part of the healing process of the partner, and laying a foundation upon which trust can be rebuilt. The therapist guides the sex addict through disclosure preparation in the weeks prior to arrival at our center. Usually the same therapist works with both the sex addict and the partner throughout the Intensive, following the procedure described below.

An alternative is to work with one person in one or two individual therapy sessions per week over an extended period in preparation for the disclosure. Concurrently, another therapist prepares the partner to receive the disclosure. After preparation is completed, we coordinate the schedules of the couple and therapists, typically blocking out half of a day for the process. A polygraph examiner is scheduled to arrive and conduct a polygraph exam immediately following the disclosure. The use of polygraph exams is covered in Chapter 9.

On the day of the disclosure, each partner meets with his or her therapist for final preparations. For the partner, this is a time to make sure he or she is in an open frame of mind and is ready to hear whatever is disclosed. She or he is reminded to listen during the disclosure without interrupting or asking questions.

The therapist may ask the partner to prepare a list of questions to ask following the disclosure. These may be questions about unexplained absences, missing money, suspicious behavior, secretive actions, or questions that have been previously asked but that yielded unsatisfactory answers. We will look at this more later in this chapter.

For the addict, the time just prior to the disclosure is used to practice reading the disclosure document, which is prepared in advance. Even though he or she has read previous versions of the disclosure aloud to the therapist over the past several weeks, this last time is more of a dress rehearsal. When it comes time for the formal disclosure, often addicts find themselves far more emotional than they anticipated and may have difficulty starting to read.

This is also a time to prepare the sex addict to listen to the questions and expressions of pain and anger from the partner that usually follow a disclosure. He or she is taught to use a good internal listening boundary, following a model developed by Pia Mellody in *Facing Codependence*,[21] to learn to let in the truth his or her partner speaks and to learn how to keep from letting in words meant only to hurt or words that are not true. For example, addicts are taught to let in reactions like "You have no idea how much you hurt me!" but to mentally block statements such as "You have never loved me!" The former is an expression of hurt, whereas the latter is intended more to inflict hurt.

When the disclosure session begins, the partner may select any seat in the room where she or he will be most comfortable. The addict is instructed to sit across the room, facing the partner. Next the therapists (if there are two) locate their seats across from each other, so that, if the members of the couple might sit at the nine o'clock and three o'clock positions, then the therapists would sit at the twelve o'clock and six o'clock positions. Chairs are arranged so that the couple is sitting about six to ten feet apart. If the partner prefers, she or he is welcome to ask the therapist to sit closer to feel more support during the disclosure session.

Once the couple is in place, one of the therapists reads the following statement:

> *The disclosure process has several parts. Those parts include reading the disclosure, processing what was heard, drafting the questions that will be asked in the polygraph exam, taking the polygraph exam, and finally the polygraph report session. New information will likely be learned today. And sometimes there is additional information that comes out in each of the parts of the disclosure process. The purpose of this process is to put an end to all secrets. The goal for the recovering sex addict is to make a permanent break with his or her acting-out behaviors. The goal of the partner is to get the truth about the spouse's behaviors so that he or she does not have to imagine what sexual things may have taken place. For the couple, the goal is to lay a foundation upon which trust can be rebuilt.*

> *(To the injured partner) This disclosure is different from a conversation that the two of you would have if you were alone. It does not contain any feelings, apology, words of love, or alibis for past behavior. Certainly we hope and believe that your spouse does love you, regrets his or her actions, and truly wants to be forgiven by you. However, we don't want any of these things to distract you from getting in touch with your feelings over what you hear in the disclosure. Hopefully, forgiveness will come and there will be a*

restoration of intimacy and relationship. That time is in the future and not something that is expected or even appropriate today. Please listen to the disclosure without any interruption. After your partner finishes reading the disclosure, you may ask any questions that you like and respond verbally any way you wish. It is also all right for you to remain silent if you so choose. Following the disclosure you will have some time with your therapist to begin to process your feelings, and then you will have the opportunity to come back and say anything additional you may wish to say.

Do either of you have any questions before the disclosure begins?

During the reading of the disclosure, the partner's therapist takes general notes to be used later to help the partner process what has been disclosed. It may be difficult for the sex addict to read the disclosure. A significant number of addicts have to stop during the disclosure to gather their emotions and recompose themselves. Partners are instructed during preparation for this session not to be distracted by any tears, even if they have never before seen the addict cry. Before beginning, the addict has been instructed to read the disclosure directly to his or her partner and to be in touch with feelings, but not to do or say anything that would be construed as a plea for sympathy.

After the disclosure is read, the partner has a chance to ask any questions that he or she wishes and to express any feelings generated by the disclosure. Usually about half of the partners have nothing to say at this time. Often they are stunned by what they have heard and need time to process it.

At this point, the therapists take the addict and the partner into individual therapy sessions. Each of them needs to be allowed to begin to process the experience and talk about his or her feelings. The task of the partner's therapist is to help her or him think through what has been disclosed. Frequently there are questions about the timeline of what occurred. During this session the partner can look through the actual disclosure document if she or he wants to. This is helpful, especially for persons who are more responsive to the eye than to the ear. It is also essential for the partner to be able to get in touch with her or his feelings during this session. The therapist can help the partner focus on the impact that hearing the disclosure had on her or him. Additionally, the partner is encouraged to express anger, sadness, or whatever emotions are present for her or him.

After both have had time with their individual therapists, all four persons get back together in the room where the disclosure took place. The partner usually has a list of questions for clarification that were prepared in the individual session. The partner asks questions, and the addict is encouraged to answer truthfully and completely and without minimizing or trying to manage the partner's response. At the end of the questioning period, the partner can freely express whatever feelings of anger or other emotions that are present.

After the partner is finished with the questions and whatever else he or she has to say, the polygraph questions are crafted. This involves both therapists and the partner. The sex addict is not part of this process. The polygraph examiner informs the sex addict of the specific questions prior to taking the exam. Suggested questions are included in the next chapter.

New information may be revealed throughout the process and even up to the polygraph exam. Our clients are instructed that if they remember anything else while they are preparing to take the polygraph exam, they must tell the examiner that they have remembered some new detail. This will be included in the report to the therapists. In that way the addict is able to express the final details and pass the exam to verify he or she has no more secrets. Any additional information that is disclosed to the polygraph examiner is revealed by the addict to the partner during the report session.

Sex addicts share a belief that if their partners knew everything they have done, they would not love them. This belief causes some individuals to hold back secrets until the very last moment. Even if this happens, the partner is prepared prior to the disclosure for the possibility that additional information may come out at any time during the process.

What Are the Benefits of Disclosure?

The research study by Schneider, Corley, and Irons[22] of sex addicts and their partners asked if they felt disclosure was an appropriate step for them. Sixty percent of addicts initially felt that disclosure was the proper course. Later in recovery, 96 percent of addicts felt disclosure was the right course of treatment for them. And in the same study, even with the pain and the trauma experienced by the partner, 81 percent of partners initially felt disclosure was the proper course of action, and in later reflection, 96 percent felt that it was the right thing to do.

The process of disclosure can provide important benefits for the spouse/partner, who finally hears the truth. The partner is reminded that he or she did not imagine the acting-out behavior. Empowerment comes with that knowledge. The partner is able to make healthy choices based on the truth.

Shameful behavior exposed to the light loses its power. The process helps sex addicts draw a line in the sand from which they can move forward, greatly increasing the possibility of living the rest of their lives free from destructive sexual behavior. Disclosure has made it possible for them to share the most shameful secrets of their addictive past. This is an important step toward restoring personal integrity. The sex addict has discovered that he or she can tell the truth, even if the truth is not pleasant.

There are also important benefits for the relationship. Disclosure allows couples to move into a new relationship, one not dominated by secrets. Once the secrets are gone, the couple has the opportunity to develop true intimacy. Disclosure provides a foundation for continued recovery. It provides a base upon which trust and intimacy can be built.

The Most Important Component of Recovery

Disclosures are important for both the partner and the sex addict. Partners have a right to know about their intimate companion's acting-out behavior. The partner's health may be at risk because of the behavior of the sex addict. And even if the addict is not directly acting out with other people, the partner still has a right to know if he or she is involved in sexual behavior that inherently has negative impacts on the relationship. Partners of sex addicts are often validated and empowered by disclosures. Upon hearing a disclosure, a partner may say, "I knew it wasn't all in my head. I am not crazy after all. My suspicions were right on target!"

While some therapists believe the greatest value of the disclosure is to the partner, and perhaps the primary purpose for a disclosure is for the partner to have information, there is also great benefit to the addict. Many who slip or have never been able to establish long-term sexual sobriety have never given a full disclosure. Deep examination reveals that there are secrets they have buried and committed to taking to their grave. Secrets have shame attached to them. Where there are secrets and shame, active addiction can find a foothold to return. The importance of getting out *all* of the secrets is discussed in the chapter on polygraph exams.

Sex addiction lives and thrives in the darkness of denial and deceit. A disclosure brings all of the secret behavior into the light. Once in the light, sex addiction loses much of its power. When sex addicts make a disclosure to their spouses or significant others, they take a major step toward restoring their integrity. The secrets they kept reinforced the feeling that they are "bad" and continued to strengthen negative thoughts about themselves. Walking in truth is fundamental to recovery from any form of addiction.

Timing

A disclosure is planned as early in the recovery process as is practical and therapeutically appropriate based on the readiness of the addict and the partner. Once it is scheduled, it usually takes several weeks to prepare both the addict and the partner for it. There are several prerequisites to disclosure. First, the addict must have made a conscious decision to stop all acting-out behavior. A disclosure done prematurely succeeds only in needlessly traumatizing the partner. Whenever possible, it is advisable to schedule a disclosure after the sex addict has a good foundation in recovery and knows what will be required in the long term.

There are circumstances where disclosure should be placed on the fast track and completed as soon as possible. If there is the potential for the partner to be exposed to a sexually transmitted disease or there are other health risks, it is crucial that the disclosure take place without delay. It is also important to proceed immediately with a disclosure if family members are involved in the addict's behavior (e.g., incest, molestation, rape).

In cases where there are children involved or who may be at risk, the disclosure should also be scheduled right away. When children are involved, it is vital for the addict to understand that the behaviors *must* be reported by the therapist to authorities as required by law and ethical mandate. The involvement of children necessitates shifting priorities to make sure that the children have adequate protection and support before focusing on other recovery issues.

Additionally, if the addict's behavior involves someone the partner knows, the disclosure should be scheduled as soon as possible. The spouse or intimate companion has a right to know without any delay if his or her partner is acting out sexually with a friend, an acquaintance, or someone at work.

Preparation of the Partner

In all cases, prior to a disclosure the partner should be in therapy with a psychotherapist skilled in working with partners of sex addicts. Psychotherapeutic support is crucial before, during, and after disclosures. The focus of this therapy is multifaceted. First, the therapist will help the partner gain an understanding of sex addiction and realize that the sex addict acts out because of the addiction and not from a lack of love or respect for his or her partner.

The therapist will also help the wounded partner understand that the sex addiction is not caused by him or her. This is an important message, because the partner may have been told repeatedly that the reason his or her spouse acts out is because he or she is not sexy enough, is overweight, does not satisfy the partner's sexual desires, or other invalid reasons. Regardless of the partner's behavior or any deficiencies, his or her behavior did not cause the addiction. A careful examination of a sex addict's behavior most often reveals that the behaviors predated the relationship by years.

In preparing the partner of a sex addict for disclosure, he or she should be reminded of the high probability that additional acting out will be revealed during the disclosure. This new information may have been long hidden or it may be relatively minor details about behavior that he or she already knows. Frequently, new information surfaces during the disclosure. Therefore, the partner must be prepared to receive a jolt of revelation; the therapist's job is to support the partner through the disclosure process, no matter how unsettling it is.

If the partner has potential for self-harm or is otherwise mentally or emotionally unstable, he or she must first be stabilized before proceeding with a disclosure. It is also a good practice for disclosure to be planned after the partner has established his or her own support network. Twelve-step organizations such as COSA, S-Anon, ISA, and CODA are important sources of support for partners during the recovery journey. The support provided by group members is invaluable not only during disclosure but throughout the recovery process.

A significant objective for the spouse or loved one during this preparation phase is in the area of finances. Partners need to have an understanding of the financial position of the family and all of the assets and accounts they have. They should know the details of the couple's or family's financial obligations, and if they do not, they need to demand this information of their partner. As revelations of the addict's behavior come out, it is crucial that the partner does not agree to *any* major changes proposed by the addict, such as moving, selling the house, or significantly increasing credit card debt. The time for making financial decisions is in the future. The immediate goal of recovery is to stabilize both partners and the relationship and not to make major financial decisions.

Sex addicts confronted with evidence of their behavior may panic and start concealing financial assets. There are cases where retirement accounts were emptied, stock portfolios liquidated, savings accounts closed, or homes refinanced without the partner's knowledge. While this is not the norm, partners of addicts need to be aware of this possibility and protect themselves, including by taking legal remedies, if they suspect any financial misdeeds.

There may be a reluctance to consult an attorney at this stage for fear of causing the situation to escalate. However, if a sex addict is making financial decisions without the partner's knowledge, taking legal action is prudent and necessary. These actions do not signal an end to the relationship. Rather, the partner is merely being farsighted and being protected from irresponsible actions of the addict.

If the partner is a wife who does not work, it may be important that she consider getting a job. Unless she is prepared to manage life on her own, including the financial aspects, it will be much more difficult for her to set boundaries concerning what behavior is acceptable or unacceptable in the relationship.

One of the most important areas of empowerment comes when a person takes time to decide what is tolerable and what is intolerable in the relationship. Partners are asked if it is acceptable for their spouse to have sex with others that puts their health at risk. Is it right if partners have time for many extracurricular activities and not invest time or emotions with the family? Usually, the response is "Of course not!" Some people are put off when being asked questions that have obvious answers. As obvious as the answers may be, in practice some partners put up with bad behavior from sex addicts for years because they fear that if they object, the sex addict will end the relationship. Some relationships do not survive sex addiction. It is possible that a marriage could end when sexual acting out is exposed, and when the companion sets boundaries about what is acceptable and what is not.

Boundary setting does not cause the relationship to end. Instead, an addict may allow it to end rather than be cut off from sexual encounters. It is not reasonable for a partner to allow his or her partner to be involved in sexual activity that does not include him or her and is not part of a healthy relationship. Fidelity is a cornerstone of marriage. If the couple is not married, there are needs for trust and understanding that are essential for an intimate relationship to be maintained, and fidelity is usually a crucial part of this.

Preparing a Disclosure Step-by-Step

What is included in the disclosure? Some sex addiction therapists limit the process to include all acting-out behavior starting at the time the sex addict met his or her relationship partner. I initially followed this model, but I now believe that disclosures should cover all sexual behavior for the addict's entire life. If anything is left out, then the couple still has secrets that stand between them.

One of the most helpful things in preparing a disclosure is to construct a timeline that includes all of the major events of life. For example, a person could number the lines on a piece of paper from one through their current age. Then they would go back and add a very brief description of major events for each year. These events are not going to be part of the disclosure, but they will help in identifying when various sexual behaviors took place.

The best disclosures are written over a period of several weeks, writing for an hour or so each day. Disclosures done hurriedly over a day or two usually result in a failed polygraph exam because much tends to be left out. In my experience, the average disclosure takes about twenty hours to write if done properly. There is not one right length for a disclosure.

Most of the clients I work with have disclosures that run from twelve to twenty pages. If a disclosure is less than ten pages, I encourage clients to go back to their timeline and see what else they can recall.

The focus of the disclosure is on behaviors, not thoughts and fantasies. Specific time frames are included. For example, the admission may be: "In 2009 I went to a strip club for the first time," or "For two months in the fall of 2011 I had a virtual sexual affair on the Internet." Names of acting-out partners are not included except in cases where the spouse knows or has had any contact with the person, or the sex addict still has contact with that person, or the person is someone the sex addict works with or has worked with in the past.

Disclosures are made using "I" statements so that the addict takes responsibility for all of his or her behaviors. For example, the sex addict should say, "I picked up a prostitute and had intercourse with her," rather than "A prostitute propositioned me and we had sex." While both sentences may be accurate, the focus should be on the addict owning up to all of his or her behaviors and not shifting responsibility to someone else or attempting to lessen the acting-out behavior by highlighting someone else's actions.

It is essential that the sex addict not shift the blame for his or her acting out. There may be a temptation to try to project his or her guilt onto the partner. For example, a man might say to his partner, "In August, you got mad at me so I went to a strip club and had oral sex with one of the dancers." Or a female sex addict might say to her husband, "Saturday, you got drunk and fell asleep on the sofa, so I went to a bar and met a guy and had intercourse." Regardless of the circumstances, the sex addict is the one who made a decision to act out.

Dates and details of the last time he or she was involved in each of various acting-out behaviors should be included—for example, "The last time I viewed pornography was in April of last year. The last time I had sexual intercourse with someone other than you was in February of this year." The addict should also give a list of arrests as well as any other encounters with law enforcement officers.

The disclosure should also include a complete list of gifts given and received from sexual partners or persons the addict hoped would become sexual partners. The recovering sex addict should make an itemized list of all expenditures incurred during his or her acting out plus a grand total of money spent. Included are other costs of addiction such as transportation, hotels, meals, alcohol and/or other drugs, therapy costs, legal expenses, lost business, gambling losses, and any other expenses that may be part of the addiction.

The sex addict needs to tell how he or she paid for those expenses and give details of any deceptions—for example, "I have a secret credit card and checking account," or "I have skimmed money out of our business," or "I always get my business expenses reimbursed in a separate check." The sex addict should also include a detailing of any money spent on sex partners over and above the list of gifts previously mentioned. If the sex addict has told an acting-out partner that he loved her or him, that is included, as are any plans that were made to start another marriage or to end the current marriage.

The disclosure should also include a list of all ways the addict deceived the relationship partner—for example, lying about going on business trips, deception about misuse of a company expense account, any secret stashes of money along with the source of those funds, the existence of secret post office boxes and secret email accounts, and secret cell phones along with the phone number and service provider. The sex addict should also provide a list of all screen names used on the Internet and all aliases used in acting out.

If other forms of addiction are involved, like substances or gambling, the sex addict needs to give a detailed account of those activities and tell how they related to the sexual acting out. Money spent on these other forms of addiction is included in the disclosure, as is a complete list of all money won and lost gambling and how the winnings were spent and the losses were covered.

With all of the detail in the disclosure, there are some things that are intentionally left out. Words of apology, expressions of love, alibis, and blame of the partner or other persons are avoided. Omitting expressions of love and apology are often the most difficult part of disclosure for both the sex addict and the partner. Both feel the need to hear these words that are often associated with owning up to a wrong. However, the use of apologies or words of love during a disclosure divert the partner's attention from being injured by the sexual addict's acting out. The partner needs to be able to fully feel the pain of the acting-out behavior to begin to heal from it.

Also omitted is assigning blame to any co-occurring disorders the sex addict may have been diagnosed with, such as depression or attention deficit hyperactivity disorder (ADHD). There are a number of psychopathologies that may make significant contributions to sex addiction, but the sex addict does not say anything that minimizes responsibility for his or her actions.

After the addict reviews the first draft of the disclosure, it usually needs to be rewritten, leaving out the more graphic details. This is not to hide anything, but rather to keep unnecessarily explicit details from further traumatizing the partner. However, all sexual acts are included, and when the sexual acting out is unprotected, the addict indicates that in the disclosure. (Note: In the disclosures I facilitate, I do not have addicts indicate when sexual acts *are* protected, because that language may sound like an effort to minimize the behavior.) After the disclosure is read, the partner can ask for any additional details that he or she would like to hear.

Not all sex addiction therapists agree about dealing with explicit details in a disclosure. Some feel strongly that the partner's right to know all details supersedes the value of protecting her or him from unnecessary trauma. An example of unnecessary or gratuitous detail would be the details of the specific positions involved in an acting-out incident of sexual intercourse. Also, details of conversations, how the addict was feeling during the acting out, and additional nonessential details are omitted. Such information may needlessly traumatize the partner and be unhelpful to the recovery of either partner or to the relationship.

When Is It Not Advisable to Have a Disclosure?

Some sex addicts believe they should not do a disclosure under the following conditions: if they think their partner will leave, if they believe the partner can't handle the information, if their acting out involves some behavior they consider degrading, or if their behavior involves sex with the partner's friends or family. On the contrary, disclosure should be made in *each* of these cases.

When is it inadvisable to have a disclosure? One such circumstance is if the couple is not committed to the marriage or relationship and has decided on divorce or termination of the relationship. If minds are made up that the relationship is at an end, there is little reason to continue with a disclosure to the spouse. Conducting disclosure at this point becomes additional fodder for divorce attorneys.

Another circumstance under which a disclosure may not be advisable is when the partner is terminally ill. While this must be decided on a case-by-case basis, it may be more beneficial to focus on providing as many positive memories as possible during her or his remaining time. However, I have worked with several couples where a partner was terminally ill but still wanted to have a full disclosure. In those instances, couples felt that the potential of finally developing true intimacy in a relationship without secrets was worth the trauma involved in the disclosure, no matter how little time they might have left.

What About Those Circumstances Where the Spouse Truly Does Not Want to Know What the Husband or Wife Has Done?

While sex addicts are quick to suggest this may be the case, few spouses prefer to remain in the dark. My experience has been that after partners of sex addicts who initially "don't want to know" build support networks in their own twelve-step groups and are empowered through their own therapy, most change their minds and believe that a full disclosure is important and something they want to hear. Also, prior to a disclosure, the partner does not know what she or he does not know. Imagination about what the sex addict has done fills the knowledge void. There have been several occasions after a disclosure when a partner has told me that what their spouse disclosed was not nearly as bad as what they imagined or feared.

Questions from the Partner After the Disclosure

As you, the partner, anticipate hearing the disclosure, it will be helpful for you to make a list of questions you can ask your spouse when the disclosure is completed. This list may be very long. Begin the list with questions that you have already asked but the answers to which you still wonder about. Your questions should include anything that you have wondered about or worried about concerning your partner's behavior. Include all of the things that have not made sense through the years. Ask about any suspicious behavior. Think about the times when you have gotten vague or inconsistent answers to the same questions.

If there are absences that are suspicious, make certain you ask specific questions about those instances. If there are financial irregularities, craft your questions so as to find out what is really going on with the family finances. If you have suspicions about certain people, this is the time to find out the truth. Following the disclosure, you need to be able to ask questions about anything that you like. Prior to the disclosure, you have been kept in the dark. Now is the time for you to be enlightened.

Many more questions will come to mind as you listen to the disclosure. You will be able to ask them as well. However, preparing an initial list of questions will help you move from shocked silence to being able to find your voice.

Partner's Response to Disclosure

The most common response to a formal disclosure is shock. The partner may tune out parts of the disclosure because what is revealed is too painful to accept or even hear. This is why the partner needs to have a therapist there for support and to listen for details that she or he might have missed. It is the therapist's responsibility to help the partner find her or his voice and to process the things heard during the disclosure.

Anger is another common response to disclosure. The partner may say things to the recovering addict such as "How could you?" or "You had no right to put my health at risk for the sake of your own enjoyment!" Anger needs to be expressed and channeled properly. A therapist is helpful in providing guidance in how to express anger in appropriate and healthy ways.

Sadness is also typical for people to express in response to disclosure. A person may feel that the entire relationship was a lie and that he or she was never truly loved. In his or her sadness the person may want to withdraw and not have any communication with the addict for a while. The range of responses to disclosure may be similar to the stages of grief. These five stages are commonly articulated as denial, anger, bargaining, depression, and acceptance. People confronted with their partner's acting out grieve for the death of a relationship, or at least for the death of what they believed their relationship to be.

One response that should be absent at the presentation of a formal disclosure of either male or female sex addicts is forgiveness. Forgiveness, it is hoped, will come as the sex addict makes a permanent break with his or her problematic sexual behavior. As the partner continues in therapy, he or she can find the right time and way to express forgiveness. But it is unfair and unrealistic to expect the partner of a sex addict to listen to a disclosure and be immediately forgiving. The partner must take time to process the pain and come to terms with what was revealed. This process takes months and sometimes years.

Premature forgiveness on the part of the partner may send the wrong message to the addict. It may be misconstrued by the addict to mean he or she can resume acting out without consequences to the relationship. The time for forgiveness comes later. Chapter 12 explores the subject of forgiveness more fully.

Other Post-Disclosure Reactions

Sex addicts often have a mixture of reactions after a disclosure. One feeling is that of relief. They are relieved to finally speak the secrets that they have hidden for many years. Intuitively they know that releasing the secrets has placed them on the path toward freedom.

But they also may have a feeling of impending loss. Many men have told me immediately following their disclosure that they are sure they have lost their wife. They are sure she will leave because of what she has heard.

Partners also have a mixture of feelings. As noted above, these feelings may include anger and sadness, but also fear about the future, or they may feel numb. Because of the many powerful emotions that are stirred up, it is crucial that both partners be supported by a therapist who is skilled in conducting disclosures.

To Separate or Not

Sometimes therapists recommend separation following disclosure, so a partner can have the space he or she may need to make sense of the information yielded by the disclosure and to process her or his feelings—without pressure from the addict. In most cases, however, unless there is a threat or fear of physical violence, I strongly suggest couples remain under the same roof. If the partner feels the need for additional space and time to process what has happened, I encourage him or her to live separately but in the same house. I believe an in-house separation rather than living at separate residences helps set the stage for future reconciliation.

In cases where the couple has young children, the separation may include sleeping in different beds in the same room. If the living situation allows, the couple can use separate rooms within the same house. Partners should have the option of deciding who stays in which room.

Some addicts are so dominating—verbally and/or physically—that partners must get away from them temporarily or permanently. This is especially true where a sex addict continues blaming his partner or puts pressure on her to immediately forgive or to verbalize trust. If the partner decides to separate, I suggest she or he stay with a friend or family member rather than staying by her- or himself. The support of a close friend or relative may be very beneficial during this traumatic period. Separation should not be seen as a prelude to inevitable divorce.

CHAPTER 9

POLYGRAPH EXAMS AS AN AID TO RECOVERY

It is important to clarify that polygraphs in sex addiction treatment serve an explicitly therapeutic purpose. Not only are these exams not designed to detect criminal behavior, but they are conducted in such a way as to make sure clients do not feel like criminals under interrogation. As a result, sex addiction-related polygraphs are conducted very differently from those used in the criminal justice system. They are used as a tool to help clients tell the truth rather than to catch them in a lie.

Chuck's Story

Chuck recalls having a polygraph exam when he applied for a job in a large warehouse. His experience was not good. Apparently the prospective employer was concerned with the potential for theft and asked lots of questions about Chuck's childhood, such as "Have you ever taken anything that was not yours?" and "Did you ever steal so much as a piece of gum when you were a child?" and "Are you a liar?" He remembers the polygraph examiner using a very intimidating manner. That unpleasant interrogation was on Chuck's mind as he was preparing to take the polygraph after his disclosure to his wife.

He was nervous about the experience and certain that his great discomfort and dread of the process would cause him to be so apprehensive that he would surely fail. He was surprised that he passed the polygraph exam. After it was over, the polygraph examiner explained to him that nervousness or fear of the polygraph exam would not cause false readings. As long as he told the truth, he would pass every exam.

Antonio's Story

Antonio, a consultant for a large computer company, failed his polygraph exam. In the course of his job, he traveled several days each week. Sometimes he was gone for more than a week. His wife Joanne became suspicious after finding a receipt for flowers that she knew he did not purchase for her. He dismissed it by saying that it was not his receipt. When she pointed out that it was his credit card number and his name on the receipt, he went into a rage and told her it was "all in her head" and she was being paranoid.

Joanne hired a private investigator, whose report cited evidence that Antonio had been involved with several women in multiple cities. Soon afterward, Antonio and Joanne sought the help of a sex addiction therapist. Antonio worked diligently on his disclosure over several weeks. He indicated his desire to reveal all of his secrets. It appeared he was being truthful. When the day of his disclosure came, he tearfully told his wife "everything" that he had done and went into detail about multiple relationships and how he had been deceptive.

However, when he took the polygraph exam to verify his disclosure, he failed. The questions asked of him were rather standard, including the following one: "Is there anything else about your sexual history you have not revealed to your wife?"

What Antonio did not reveal was that one of the women he was sexual with was a colleague at work. By withholding this secret, Antonio was not telling his wife the whole truth and failed his exam, losing what little trust Joanne had left. He felt he had a good reason to withhold this detail. Antonio reasoned that since the affair had ended more than a year ago, he did not want to risk his wife insisting that he make changes at work or perhaps change jobs.

Antonio's failure came from denying a fundamental truth:

A DISCLOSURE THAT IS LESS THAN 100 PERCENT HONEST AND COMPLETE IS NOT A DISCLOSURE, BUT JUST ANOTHER DECEPTION.

A person will have no difficulty passing a polygraph if his or her intention is to be completely honest and not hold back anything. Persons who hold back even small details do not have a chance of passing the exam.

Polygraph as an Aid to Disclosure

Polygraph exams are necessary to ensure that complete honesty and true recovery are taking place. In substance addiction treatment, a urinalysis is done at the beginning of treatment and randomly throughout treatment and aftercare. Urinalysis is used to verify a person's self-report and ascertain the actual status of his or her abstinence from substances. Substance addiction treatment programs frequently require such objective proof that the person remains substance-free. Polygraph exams provide verification of sex addicts' self-reports and provide more objective evidence of their abstinence from problematic sexual behavior.

Lying is necessary for sex addiction to remain hidden. The only way for a sex addict to hide his or her problematic sexual behavior is to develop advanced skills at deception and duplicity. Sex addicts can lie with such conviction that they may even convince themselves that the lies they tell are true. They may lie with impunity and do it so habitually that they may not be conscious of how often they lie.

The deceptive behavior of sex addicts is especially troublesome because some are so convincing that they can lie with tears in their eyes and tell their partner, "This is the absolute truth." After repeatedly catching a sex addict in a lie, the partner is left to wonder how he or she will ever know the truth. Mistrust and doubt undermine every aspect of a relationship, creating such insecurity that a wife may wonder, "Is he being truthful when he says he loves me?" Or the husband whose wife has repeatedly acted out and who hears her promise to be faithful may remain skeptical.

Partial disclosures traumatize the partner. Polygraphs help get to the truth. Without this procedure, many sex addicts would never be able to tell the complete truth. Unless the entire truth is disclosed, the sex addict may never be able to get free from an entrenched pattern of problematic sexual behavior.

Sex addicts lie to their partners, to their therapists, and to themselves. A research project I conducted a few years ago among sex addicts revealed that they were untruthful about many of their behaviors. A number of sex addicts responded that they had been dishonest not only with their spouses, but also with therapists. One person said, "I have lied through the years to all of my therapists. They are so gullible." Another admitted, "Therapists are so easy to fool. I just tell them what I think they want to hear."[23] I accept that I have been lied to in therapy in the past and will be lied to in the future.

I am not surprised that sex addicts lie to their therapists. Though it is disheartening that an addict would seek help for the addiction and then not be truthful about his or her behavior, dishonesty is one of the behavioral hallmarks of addiction. The nature of therapy requires a high level of trust between the client and therapist. In the absence of additional or contrary information or an implausible story, the only information therapists have to go on is what their clients share with them.

With the use of polygraph I know the truth about clients' behaviors. Just as important, spouses can be certain that the disclosure they receive in the clinical setting is complete. As one woman put it, "I can't trust my husband, but I can trust the polygraph exam!" She has a right and also the responsibility to know what her spouse has been involved in. Not only does deception keep one's spouse from finding out about the problematic sexual behavior, it is often part of the defense mechanism addicts use in order to live with their addictive behaviors. Sex addicts may lie to themselves about the impact of their behavior on their lives and their families. They may even have some success convincing themselves that they were justified in their sexual dalliances.

Polygraph exams break through the deception and lies. Not only does a polygraph exam allow spouses of sex addicts to get to the truth, the exam requires addicts to expose the layers of shame connected to their sexual acting out that are keeping them enslaved to their addiction. Polygraph exams make it possible for them to finally tell the complete truth. This may be the first time in his or her life that the sex addict has been able to be totally truthful. It should be noted that while the decision to take a polygraph exam must rest with the addict, he or she has the opportunity to raise his or her level of credibility and accountability if the disclosure is followed up with a polygraph. Once sex addicts realize that the polygraph exam is a tool for helping them get the whole truth out, most are able to be more forthright in their disclosure and expose all of the facts concerning their acting out. But if a person is intent on being deceptive, polygraph exams expose this. There are persons who hold onto a secret with the hope that they can get it by the polygraph examiner, only to fail their exam.

Today's polygraphs are highly reliable, computer-assisted tools for getting at the truth. False positives and other questionable outcomes are more a product of outdated polygraph processes than current practices.

Polygraph Protocol

The typical polygraph protocol we use allows for four relevant questions that are supplied by the therapist in consultation with the spouse. These questions are developed in session with only the partner of the sex addict present. The questions for the polygraph exam are global enough to cover the entire disclosure, and specific enough to address areas of particular concern for the spouse. Polygraph examiners will add additional questions for the purpose of validating the exam.

The following are samples of questions that may be included in an initial or baseline polygraph exam. From this list, four questions are selected. Often a partner may want to have a question addressing a specific situation that the sex addict has denied. The actual questions used will be determined by the therapist after hearing the disclosure and listening to concerns that have been expressed by the partner.

1. Is there anything about your sexual history that you have not told your partner?

2. Were you purposely deceptive in any way during the disclosure process?

3. Have you purposely omitted any sexual behavior from your disclosure?

4. Have you had physical sexual contact with any person other than what you have disclosed?

5. Have you intentionally viewed any pornography since (DATE)?

6. Have you patronized any sex-oriented businesses since (DATE)?

As you can see, several questions are similar. Careful selection and wording of questions will reveal the truthfulness (or lack thereof) of the disclosure. Specificity is important, but a greater concern is for the questions to be broad enough so that they not allow any sexual behavior to go undetected. As a rule, we use more global questions to verify that the disclosure has been complete and truthful rather than targeting specific instances of sexual behavior. However, if the spouse has one or two areas he or she is particularly concerned about, we can use one or two of the questions to delve into those concerns. For example, if, after hearing her husband's disclosure, a wife wonders if something sexual has occurred between her husband and her sister, we will ask about that specifically. The question might be worded, "Have you ever been sexual with your wife's sister?" The phrase "Have you ever been sexual" includes not only sexual acts but sexual conversations and hugs and kisses that are something more than a family greeting.

When the polygraph questions have been written, the addict goes to the polygraph examiner's office and takes the exam. The sex addict signs a release allowing the therapist to directly consult with the examiner. He or she takes the disclosure along in case there are questions about behavior in his or her past. In the meantime, the partner and the partner's therapist have another individual session to further process the events of the formal disclosure. This additional therapy time is important because the spouse has often been traumatized by what was disclosed and needs help to cope with what has transpired.

Additional information is often revealed during the polygraph exam because a sex addict may have been holding back information, hoping to slip it past the polygraph exam. But it is more likely that the added pressure of taking the exam may cause the sex addict to remember long-hidden or forgotten secrets or details.

What Happens When a Sex Addict Fails a Polygraph Exam Following a Disclosure?

Among other things, failing a polygraph exam indicates that a person needs to do additional work on his or her disclosure. What did he or she leave out? What did he or she remember but fail to write down? For the persons who say, "I have told everything that I remember" and still fail, the reality is that they have recalled something that they have chosen not to reveal. Some secrets are buried so deeply or have such shame attached to them that it is extremely difficult for sex addicts to summon the courage to disclose them.

After working more on the disclosure, the sex addict has an opportunity to take another polygraph exam. In my practice I have rarely seen addicts fail a second exam if they reveal what they left out during their first exam.

What Should the Partner's Response Be if the Sex Addict Fails a Polygraph Exam?

The first response should be to reserve judgment. Realize that it is a very difficult process for sex addicts to stop a lifelong habit of lying and suddenly tell the whole truth. The belief that they may lose their relationship if they are candid about their behavior is a powerful incentive to hide the truth.

Every time I have had clients fail an exam, they act surprised and claim to have no idea why they failed. They may blame the failure on being nervous or not being liked by the polygraph examiner, or just say that the results are wrong. But in virtually all of these instances, eventually additional information came out allowing them to take and pass a second exam. And in those rare cases where they fail a second exam, usually between the work of the therapist and the partner who has been empowered by objective evidence of the sex addict's continued deception, the final secrets are revealed.

The purpose of the polygraph as I use it is to help sex addicts tell the complete truth. A failed exam is an indicator that there is something else that the sex addict is afraid to disclose. Often it is these last secrets that keep a person bound to his or her addiction. Therapists can work with the sex addict and the partner to create a safe place for the truth to be told, allowing for a foundation upon which trust can be built so that the relationship can be put back on track. Once the addict's most hidden secrets are revealed, he or she can begin dealing with the shame that has accompanied those secrets. The release of the secrets is a predicate for releasing the shame.

But there are still sex addicts who will stubbornly maintain that they are telling the truth and that there is something wrong with the results. Certainly any decision the partner makes is her or his own. He or she needs to work with a therapist to determine what is in his or her best interest as well as the interest of any children who may be living at home. At this point, some individuals experience a boundary collapse and decide that they want to hold onto the relationship at any cost, even in the face of their spouse's continued deception and acting out. Whatever the choice, the partner should make decisions only after exploring all alternatives.

Parker's Story

Parker agreed to do a full disclosure to his partner Kacee. He also knew his therapist was going to encourage him to take a polygraph exam to verify that he had been truthful about his disclosure and had not left anything out. The disclosure revealed many additional things that Kacee did not know, and she was devastated by the information. When Parker took his polygraph exam, the questions focused on whether he had been truthful in the disclosure and whether he omitted any behavior. He failed his exam. While he swore he was telling the truth and that there must be some problem with the polygraph process, Kacee did not believe him. Parker was even tearful in pleading his case, pointing out that if he had intended to intentionally lie, he would not have revealed many of the things that were included in the disclosure.

Parker's therapist was skilled in sex addiction therapy and did not use the failed test to badger Parker, but rather pointed out that it might be possible that there was either some event in his past that was so shameful that he could not bring himself to reveal it or there was a behavior that he felt Kacee would not be able to forgive. Parker committed to continuing work with his therapist to see if there was something else in his background that he was either consciously or subconsciously holding back. After several sessions he finally told his therapist that there was one additional thing he had not revealed, and that was a recent relationship he had had with a fellow employee. He also felt that this last bit of information would cause Kacee to leave him. After revealing this last detail, Parker took and passed another polygraph exam, verifying that there were no other hidden behaviors. Ultimately Parker and Kacee stayed together, but he opted to get a job with a different company so that he did not continue a close working relationship with his former sex partner.

There are several reasons a person may fail a polygraph exam. One reason that must be dealt with up front is the margin of error that is inherent in all diagnostic processes such as medical exams. Current polygraph exams have a 94 percent-plus accuracy rate. Sex addicts who fail exams may be quick to suggest that they are truthful and that the exams are inaccurate. After doing additional therapy, if the client maintains that there is nothing new to disclose, I offer him or her the opportunity to take another exam and even offer the opportunity to use a different examiner. Two exams with the same questions but utilizing different examiners virtually negates any margin of error.

In the event that the addict fails a second polygraph exam, I encourage a partner to give him or her some additional latitude and to continue working with the partner's own therapist to get the truth into the open. After additional work on the disclosure to uncover any additional details that have been hidden, the sex addict has an opportunity to take a subsequent exam. The goal is to help the addict to be completely honest and allow the partner to get to the truth. The partner needs to remember that this process is not meant to find a reason to get out of the relationship, but rather to get to the complete truth.

He or She Passed the Polygraph Exam: Now What?

Following the polygraph exam, the couple and both therapists reconvene for the polygraph report session. In some cases there are additional details that have come to light, and these will need to be talked about at length. The sex addict is the one who gives these additional details to his or her partner. Sometimes no additional details are revealed. When this is the case the report session becomes anticlimactic, but this is still an important component in the process.

I opt not to get a written report from the polygraph examiner. I have found that a verbal report can be much more detailed. Ultimately, the information I need from the examiner is whether the person passed or failed the exam. Sometimes a written report can become ammunition for some future argument.

Passing their polygraph exams following formal disclosure is such a momentous event for sex addicts that they often feel as if they should be congratulated for telling the truth. Certainly, it is a laudable accomplishment for them to be able to make a break with their long-standing habit of telling lies and to finally reveal the complete truth. During the next several days after passing the polygraph exam, the partner may want to express appreciation for the addict's telling the truth and perhaps for having had the courage to take that step. But the self-vindication and exuberance often displayed by the sex addict in the aftermath of a polygraph exam that verifies the disclosure stands in stark contrast to the anger and/or sadness that the partner feels after learning the details of the sexual acting out. The partner should allow her- or himself the freedom to feel the full range of emotions and express them to the addict. The best place to do this is in a clinical setting with therapists present. The partner needs to have the opportunity to express whatever emotions are felt.

The partner's therapist will help her or him to understand the importance of expressing her or his emotions, and the addict's therapist will help the sex addict prepare to listen without retreating into shame or defensiveness. It is appropriate for the addict to feel guilt over the acting-out behavior, but it is not helpful to plunge into shame. Guilt is awareness that he or she did some things that were wrong. Shame is the sex addict seeing himself or herself as an inherently bad person.

Misuse of Polygraph Exams

Polygraph exams should be used as a part of the process of recovery from sex addiction *only* if they are an integrated part of therapy. Great harm has been done when a couple has engaged a polygraph examiner directly without utilizing the skills and expertise of a trained sex addiction therapist familiar with integrating polygraph into the therapeutic process.

There have been cases where additional acting out and secrets were revealed after a person had taken and passed a polygraph exam. In each case, the exams that were administered did not follow a clinical disclosure, but rather asked nonspecific questions concerning whether the addict has revealed all of his or her sexual behavior *or* the questions were so specific that they did not cover the sex addict's entire sexual history. The false assurance given by an erroneous exam impedes sex addiction recovery because the addict still has secrets that will likely lead him or her back into addiction.

Additionally, most polygraph examiners are well versed in using exams in criminal proceedings. They may conduct them for the police and for attorneys to find out if a person has engaged in criminal activity. They may even use them with sex offenders to verify that they have not reoffended while on probation. But the use of polygraph exams in sex addiction therapy is very different. The person being tested is not a criminal and should not be treated as one. Polygraph exams should not be used in a punitive way or as a way of gathering evidence on someone suspected of being unfaithful. For that reason it is necessary for the therapist to work closely with the polygraph examiner and develop a procedure that treats the addict with the utmost respect and without any of the overtones of a criminal procedure. Polygraph exams that are part of sex addiction recovery therapy are used as an aid to the addict to help strip away all of the layers of deception that have been used to facilitate the addiction.

If a sex addict really believes his partner will leave him, he will likely try to protect secrets as long as possible. The fact that he is engaged in sex addiction therapy that includes a disclosure and polygraph is evidence of motivation to get rid of all of his secrets. It takes a patient and supportive therapist to guide this difficult process, even if it means doing additional disclosure and a follow-up test after failure of the first polygraph exam. An initial exam failure is not final for the individual. Instead, it is an indication that further work needs to be done to get to the bottom of the secrets so that the addict can finally get free.

It is tempting for some couples to use polygraph exams for settling arguments or validating the assertions of the sex addict. He or she may say, "I can prove to you that I'm telling the truth. I'll go take a polygraph exam!" Or the partner may exclaim, "I don't believe you. You need to take a polygraph exam."

To use polygraph in this way is misuse of a valuable tool. It is also a misuse of polygraph exams at the beginning of recovery to "out" the sex addict simply as a means of determining whether the partner wants to stay in the marriage. Polygraph exams are helpful for verifying a clinically facilitated and supervised disclosure and for monitoring continued progress in recovery. Couples should resist the urge to use polygraph capriciously or punitively. Instead, the couple should be content with a previously agreed-upon schedule for follow-up exams. Follow-up exams and a schedule for aftercare work are discussed in Chapter 16.

CHAPTER 10

THE PARTICULARS OF POLYGRAPH USE IN SEX ADDICTION THERAPY

Karl's Story

Karl and Mattie had looked forward to their intensive outpatient treatment program since they had signed up for it three months before. While they waited for their intensive treatment, Mattie had Karl take a polygraph exam because she was concerned that he was having an affair with someone he worked with.

When they started their Intensive, Karl proudly told the therapist that he had already passed a polygraph exam and was sure he would not have a problem passing the exam that followed his disclosure. However, he failed that exam. He claimed he did not know why he failed the exam. As he thought about it, he said he was sure that it was probably because there were so many things that he had done in his life that he could not remember them all. The results of his failed exam empowered Mattie. She'd suspected there was something else that he was not telling; now she knew.

Even though Karl claimed he did not know why he failed, his therapist explained to him that he did not fail because of what he could not remember. Rather, he failed because there were other behaviors that he had engaged in that he did not disclose to his wife.

Before his treatment program concluded, Karl admitted to Mattie that he was indeed having an affair. It was with a neighbor. With his additional disclosure, he took another polygraph exam and this time easily passed.

How did Karl pass the polygraph exam he took prior to his disclosure? He was asked specific questions about unfaithfulness with a particular person. And that first exam was not intended to confirm a clinical disclosure. The questions Mattie was interested in were too narrowly focused. The mistake Karl and Mattie made was in believing that what would fix their relationship was a passed polygraph exam. Actually, what they needed was to be guided through a formal disclosure and rebuilding process by a sex addiction therapist who then used polygraph as a part of therapy.

Sometimes in the criminal justice system polygraph exams may be seen as an adversarial process, but in sex addiction therapy I view polygraph as a collaboration among the therapist, the client, the client's partner, and the polygraph examiner. I view the examiner as part of the treatment team in helping people get free from their problematic sexual behaviors. Polygraph is used in my practice as an integrated part of therapy with sex addicts and their partners. Polygraph exams are used initially to verify that a clinical disclosure is truthful and complete. Then they are used periodically as part of a rigorous aftercare process to verify that old behaviors have not recurred and that there are not any new acting-out behaviors.

During our Three-Day Intensives, polygraph exams are used in the same manner but scheduled a bit differently. Clinical disclosures take place on the first day, and then the sex addict has that evening to review his or her disclosure to see if he or she can recall any additional details. Then polygraph exams are scheduled for the second day of the Intensive. Usually we give the results to the couple immediately after the exam is completed.

Interview with a Polygraph Examiner

The following is an interview with polygraph examiner Stephen Cabler.[24] Mr. Cabler has been the primary polygraph examiner for Hope & Freedom Counseling Services for the past several years.

Magness: How many polygraph exams have you conducted?

Cabler: Somewhere over 7,000.

Magness: I know when we first started working together, you said you had not used polygraph in working closely with a therapist.

Cabler: That's right.

Magness: How many sex addiction–related exams have you now conducted?

Cabler: You and I now average three exams a week. We have done about 750 exams together. In addition to that, I now work with twenty-four other therapists who focus on sex addiction. I have done another 175 to 200 exams for them.

Magness: How are polygraph exams that are supportive of sex addiction therapy similar to other exams?

Cabler: They are similar in that they are used to find out if a person is telling the truth or being deceptive. Both involve questions, the polygraph instrument, and me interpreting the results.

Magness: How do these exams differ from other exams that you conduct?

Cabler: Polygraphs for sex addiction are not criminal in nature. We work hard to make sure clients do not feel like criminals when we work with them, so I conduct these differently than when I am doing an exam for the criminal justice system. And I want them to know that I am interested in helping them tell the truth.

Magness: You mentioned the criminal justice system. I didn't think polygraph exams could be used in court.

Cabler: That's not right. They are not used to introduce or corroborate direct evidence in court. However, I testify in court frequently about the criminal exams that I conduct. Judges also have the prerogative of ordering witnesses and potential witnesses to take a polygraph exam.

Magness: Please tell me more about how they are used in the legal system.

Cabler: If the police have a suspect that they believe has committed a crime, they may give that person the opportunity to take a polygraph exam to prove his innocence. And there are several other instances where I work with attorneys who use polygraph exams to add weight to their client's innocence in preparing a grand jury packet that is used to determine whether or not there is sufficient evidence to go to trial.

Magness: And then there is the use of polygraphs in the probation and parole system.

Cabler: Right. Polygraph exams are used to determine if a person who is on probation or parole has complied with the terms of their release. I have found judges put great weight on the results of those exams. Failing an exam can lead to a person having their parole or probation revoked.

Magness: Let's get back to the differences in exams that are part of the criminal justice system and those that are used to support sex addiction therapy.

Cabler: Criminal justice–related exams are very specific in that they relate to a specific target issue. These exams are conducted to help determine a person's truthfulness about a very specific single incident or act.

Magness: So then sex addiction–related exams are broader?

Cabler: Yes. Exams that back up a clinical disclosure cover a broad period of time. When a disclosure is thorough, it covers the entire sexual history of a person all the way up to the time of the polygraph exam.

Magness: I want to go back to the interview phase of the exam. What do you look for when you are asking a client questions about their disclosure?

Cabler: Well, the first thing I want to do is to make sure I understand what the client has said in his disclosure.

Magness: You said his. Are your clients only men?

Cabler: No. But most of the sex addiction exams that I have conducted have been on men. There have also been women who struggle with sex addiction that I have tested.

Magness: So you make sure you understand the disclosure. What do you do then?

Cabler: I look for gaps. I have done enough of these exams now that the areas of potential gaps jump out at me. I look for periods of no sexual acting out and attempt to verify that indeed no acting out was taking place at that time. I also ask questions, based on my experience with disclosures, to see if there are other behaviors present.

Magness: Stephen, we have slowly refined our process over the past several years. I know what both of us want is for each person tested to pass his or her exam.

Cabler: We actually tell clients that we not only want them to pass but that we will do everything we can to help them pass. And the way to help them to pass is to encourage them to tell the complete truth.

Magness: How is it possible to help someone pass an exam?

Cabler: The first thing is in the purpose of the exam. It is not in anyone's best interest to come to the end of an exam and have to tell the client and his partner that he failed, that he was deceptive. I see my job as that of helping the client tell the truth. I assume that he wants to and that is why he has agreed to be tested. So my job then is to help him get the whole truth out. I want to help him fill in any gaps that might exist in the disclosure that he has given to his partner during therapy.

Magness: How do you do that?

Cabler: That is part of the interview process that happens prior to running the charts.

Magness: Assume for a moment that I do not know anything about polygraph exams. Tell me what happens during a polygraph exam.

Cabler: The testing process is in three phases. The first phase is the information-gathering phase. There are a number of forms that the client fills out where I get some basic history and review any medical issues that might impact the exam. This phase also includes a thorough interview where I review the disclosure that the examinee read to his therapist and to his wife.

I use my experience to recognize places that seem out of the norm or if something is missing and continue asking questions until I feel I have exhausted my ability to detect that more needs to be said. At that point it is time to rely on the polygraph equipment, which begins phase two. After the charts (which indicate the results) have been run and evaluated and the results determined, then it is time for phase three of the polygraph, which is the post-test interview. If the examinee passes, the post-test interview is obviously short; if the person does not pass, then a second interview ensues. Many therapists want to give the results in therapy so both partners get the results together. In those cases the therapist conducts the post-test interview.

Magness: Why is the interview process necessary?

Cabler: The interview process is where I review the details of the disclosure with the client. Usually the client signs a release with the therapist so that the therapist can share with me any information that came out during the disclosure. Clients also bring their written disclosure with them to the exam.

Magness: So does the client read the disclosure to you like he did with the therapist?

Cabler: Not usually. Normally, I will ask questions based on what I read in the disclosure notes supplied to me by the therapist.

Magness: Isn't that what has just taken place in the therapist's office?

Cabler: It is certainly similar. But as you have heard me say several times, I'm not a therapist. So my questions about the disclosure may come from a different perspective than that of a therapist.

Magness: Do you ever have clients give you additional information during the interview process?

Cabler: That happens quite often.

Magness: Does that cause a person to fail an exam?

Cabler: Actually, just the opposite happens. Sometimes it is difficult for a person to give up those last secrets. He may have a lot of shame and is reluctant to let go of those secrets. But if he can give up all of his secrets and be completely truthful, then we can exclude those things from the exam and test the person to see if he is now being truthful.

Magness: What happens to additional information that comes out during an exam?

Cabler: It becomes part of the report that I give to the therapist.

Magness: You mentioned a report. Is this a written report?

Cabler: As you know, I used to always give you a written report of the exam. But as we refined our process, we have found that there are several advantages to making this report a verbal report.

Magness: What are those advantages?

Cabler: Well, in the exams that we do together, I am able to give a much more thorough report when I do it orally and I am able to do this immediately after the exam without having to wait until I can produce a written report. We typically spend an extended period of time together reviewing the results of the exam. We talk about the individual questions that were asked as well as any new information that came out during the interview. I know I have had some clients tell me things they were reluctant to say in front of their wife and therapist. I review that in detail with you or the other therapists I work with.

Magness: Are there other advantages to not using a written report?

Cabler: There is a significant time advantage. If I do a written report, it takes me another couple of hours to prepare that report. And if I do not have to prepare a written report, I am able to keep my fees lower than they might be otherwise.

Magness: Tell me more about the second phase of the exam.

Cabler: That is when I review the questions that are going to be asked on the exam and then run the charts; that is, I ask the client the questions and the polygraph records the physiological responses. I make sure the client knows the questions that are going to be asked so there are no surprises during the exam. The client is hooked up to the polygraph apparatus and I ask the questions that were provided by the therapist. I also add additional questions that are designed to make sure I get the whole truth on the exam.

Magness: You run more than one chart; that is, you ask the questions more than once?

Cabler: According to rules and regulations governing polygraph exams, there must be a minimum of two charts run in order to render a decision, and there can be no more than five.

Magness: Why not just ask the questions once?

Cabler: This is to ensure that we get reliable results. For example, if I run one chart and get a significantly higher reading on a question than I anticipated, I then run additional charts to see if I get the same results or if that was just an anomaly. In polygraph, one of the important things we pay attention to is consistencies and inconsistencies of responses to questions asked. Nothing can be determined from a question that was asked only one time.

Magness: So if you don't get the same high reading on the other charts, will the client fail because of the high reading on the one chart?

Cabler: No. That is because I am able to show that the response was out of the ordinary and then verify by running additional charts in which the person's physiology did not indicate deception. But it is not as simple as giving a higher or lower response physiologically. There are several different criteria that we observe in each component used to detect deception. These are compared one to the other after the questions have been asked multiple times, and we also move the questions around as far as their order.

Magness: How reliable are polygraph exams?

Cabler: I am not in the research area, but studies that have been conducted by the Department of Defense have shown polygraph exams to be 85 to 90 percent accurate or greater.

Magness: So that means ten to fifteen of every hundred exams are wrong?

Cabler: No, it doesn't. It is not just about numbers. First of all, that is for all exams that are conducted with all examiners. Remember that this 10 to 15 percent also includes inconclusive results, which actually make up the majority of those percentages. Inconclusive results are due to many reasons—for example, illegal drug use, undiagnosed mental illness, or a person who purposely tries to make himself untestable by not following the simple instructions given during the exam. Most of these occurrences happen during criminal polygraphs where a suspect is intent on being deceptive.

Magness: I assume that the training and expertise of the examiner have a bearing on the validity of an exam.

Cabler: Certainly. I'm sure it is just like therapists; some are better than others.

Magness: How confident are you in the results of the exams that we conduct together?

Cabler: I am as close to 100 percent sure of the results as I can be.

Magness: How can you be so confident?

Cabler: Well, first of all, the process that is used with sex addiction therapy is different from what is used for any other exam. We have clients who are voluntarily coming to us for help to get free from their problem behaviors. The therapist does a methodical job of helping the client put together a complete disclosure. Before I ever see a client, I know their disclosure has been carefully examined. Then the therapist identifies any areas that they are concerned about. In addition to that, the partner and the therapist carefully craft the questions for the exam. Then my interview typically approaches the disclosure from a different perspective that helps to surface anything that the client may have forgotten.

Magness: Or intentionally left out?

Cabler: Certainly that happens. But I try to help the clients get rid of their secrets. It is my job to help them tell the truth. Based on my experience with many clients, I know it may be very difficult for them to get the whole truth out. But getting the truth out helps to set them free.

Magness: I know we had one client who told us he didn't value polygraph because he said he had lied on an exam he took that asked him if he cheated on a fishing tournament.

Cabler: Yes, but since we were not there and don't know the complete circumstances of that exam, we don't know how the exam was conducted and what questions were asked. But I also know that I was approached by a very large fishing organization and asked to provide polygraph services for each of their upcoming tournaments. They told me they wanted me to use the same process they used for years and just line up all of the winners and give them a quick test that didn't take longer than thirty minutes each. I declined the work. It is not possible to give a valid test in that short a period of time. So if that is the type of exam that he was given, I am not surprised at those results.

Magness: How long does it take to conduct a proper exam?

Cabler: It generally takes about two hours, but sometimes they may take longer. All polygraph exams are different. I have exams that are complete in an hour and I have exams that have gone three hours. A sex addiction full disclosure exam will on an average take me a minimum of two hours. I have learned a lot about sex addiction and I know where I need to hunt for information after reading a disclosure.

Magness: For the person who has never taken a polygraph exam, can you tell them a little bit about the experience?

Cabler: Sure. The first thing a client notices is the special chair that is used for the exams. It is constructed so as to help facilitate the best possible results. Next there are two pneumograph tubes, one placed around the lower abdomen and the other across the upper chest area. A cardio cuff is placed around the bicep area of the arm, and the last component, known as the electrodermal response electrodes, are two probes that are attached to the tips of the fingers. During the exam the cardio cuff is inflated to roughly 60 to 80 psi for the entire time the charts are running, which may average about four minutes per chart. Sometimes there are additional measurements taken as part of the exam.

Magness: How does the polygraph work?

Cabler: There are physiological changes that take place when a person is deceptive. These are very small, almost imperceptible changes. However, they are measurable. The polygraph measures and records these changes in a person's physiology. Polygraph examiners are trained to read these charts and interpret the results.

Magness: I had a polygraph examiner tell me that he needed to intimidate people during the exam to get the results he wanted. Is that true?

Cabler: I don't believe in intimidation. In fact the use of intimidation can result in a false positive. I never intimidate a client. I want to help the clients relax so that they are comfortable and are willing to tell me the truth. I can't scare or bully a person into telling the truth. But if a person wants to get honest, I can help them do that.

Magness: I have heard of people trying to use techniques to beat a polygraph exam. Is that possible?

Cabler: You are talking about countermeasures. Among polygraph examiners we get amused at some of the things that people try to use to beat an exam. Those are things that have been around for many years and are not effective in beating a modern digital polygraph exam. And besides, an attempt to use countermeasures is easy to spot, and that results in an automatic fail. A person attempting to use countermeasures is being deceptive, so the results of the exam are "Deception indicated."

Magness: I remember we had a man who was trained in the military special forces and said he was taught how to beat a polygraph exam.

Cabler: And as I recall, he failed his exam.

Magness: He did fail his first one. Then he eventually revealed his complete history to his wife and passed a second exam.

Magness: I know you are licensed by the state. How often do you have to renew your license?

Cabler: I renew it every year. And I typically take twenty to forty continuing education units a year to stay competent.

Magness: Is there anything additional you would like to add before we end the interview?

Cabler: Just how gratifying my work is when I am working with sex addicts. I have found that most of them are very good people who desperately want to get free from the problem behaviors they have battled for years. I get to witness the relief that comes to clients' faces when they finally get all of their secrets out. They know they have finally gotten honest. They have gotten free. That look on their faces makes my job worthwhile.

CHAPTER 11

THE USE OF CELIBACY CONTRACTS

Julius's Story

Julius first saw pornography at age thirteen when visiting the home of a friend. His friend showed him a collection of magazines that were filled with photos of naked women. The magazines belonged to his friend's older brother. Julius experienced a strong emotional reaction from viewing the first photo. From then on he would seize any opportunity to get another look at those magazines.

He would suggest to his friend that they look at his brother's magazines each time he visited. Julius recalled his friend reacting negatively and telling him that all he wanted to do was look at those magazines. As he grew older, Julius slowly gathered his own collection of pornography. From that time on he was never without a stash of pornography.

As an adult, he bookmarked hundreds of websites where he could view pornography. He spent five hours or more each evening searching for new pornography. His search was not just for any pornography but for certain types of photos. When he found photos that he liked, he would download them and store them on his computer. Seldom would he go back and look at the photos that he downloaded, but he would continue the search for the perfect photos that fit the profile of his ideal fantasy partner. Over the past five years Julius has downloaded hundreds of thousands of photos and videos and has spent an average of thirty-plus hours each week in his cybersex behavior. By his own estimation he has spent over eight thousand hours engaged in his sex addiction in just five years. He realized that he invested time in his addiction that was almost equal to having a second full-time job. He also admitted that he used special programs to search for pornography and as a result had accumulated more than ten terabytes of pornography. This was more than he could view in a lifetime!

At the suggestion of his therapist, Julius and his partner decided to write a celibacy contract. His therapist told Julius that he believed a period of celibacy would help him to clear his mind of the many pornographic images that he had seen and help set the stage for moving into healthy sexuality with his partner later. With the establishment of the initial contract period, Julius and his partner were encouraged to see the contract as part of the treatment and recovery process, and not as punishment. As the name suggests, a celibacy contract is an agreement between the couple to forgo all sexual activity for a period *of time. Typical contracts are set for thirty days and then reviewed with the couple, with possible extensions made on a monthly basis. However, that does not mean that every couple dealing with sex addiction needs to have a celibacy contract.*

There are several advantages to a celibacy contract that may encourage a couple to consider its use. The first is that it removes the "drug of choice" from a sex addict. Sex addiction, like other manifestations of addiction, creates changes in brain chemistry and functioning. A first step in treating alcohol and other drug abuse is to take the addict completely off his or her substances so that treatment can begin and progress in an environment of abstinence. A celibacy contract has the effect of taking the sex addict off his or her "drug" and establishing that environment of abstinence.

The celibacy contract precludes not only sexual intercourse between the couple, but all sexual activity. It should also include a ban on all masturbation, use of pornography, and any other sexual behavior involving other people or oneself. If masturbation does not end, the celibacy contract is of no practical benefit.

Compulsive sexual behavior is used as a drug to take away pain, to cope with stress, to manage difficult circumstances in life, and perhaps even as a reward for some achievement. When sex is removed, addicts often have a variety of feelings and emotions surface that are unfamiliar to them, since they usually medicate themselves to keep from feeling them. During the term of a celibacy contract, addicts have a chance to get in touch with their feelings and face what they have been hiding from.

Both partners need to be in therapy for the duration of the celibacy contract so that they are able to process feelings and emotions that may be coming to the surface. Sometimes the issues that surface during this period provide significant insight into the treatment of the problematic sexual behavior. If sex has been used to solve problems or end disagreements in the relationship, the contract period will encourage couples to deal with their difficulties more directly.

The mention of a celibacy contract may bring fear to an addict. I have heard individuals, particularly men, say that they cannot even conceive of going a week without sex, to say nothing of a month or longer. If they are that dependent on sex, the celibacy contract will allow them to face some of the fears they have associated with temporary abstinence.

Partners, on the other hand, often greet the thought of a celibacy contract with a sense of relief. In some relationships, partners feel pressured to be sexual at a frequency that is far beyond their comfort zone. Also, they may dread sex because it is often one-sided, with the sex addict's appetite being the first priority and the partner's needs being marginalized.

There are several additional advantages to a celibacy contract. As mentioned earlier, it allows for the examination of feelings that may have been masked by sex. A celibacy contract allows the couple to develop a healthy sexual appetite for each other. This is especially helpful in relationships where the sex addict does not seem to have much interest in sex with his or her spouse. If he or she completely suspends sexual behavior, including all masturbation and pornography use, his or her sexual appetite has an opportunity to normalize and, it is hoped, result in a greater desire to have sex within the spousal relationship. This normalization process may require the contract to be renewed for an additional thirty to sixty days or more. This may seem like an eternity, but the renewed intimacy that can result is worth postponing sexual gratification.

Another advantage to a celibacy contract is that the period of sexual abstinence provides time for a couple to consider what kind of sexual relationship they want to have and maintain. If the relationship has included activities that either partner believes were unhealthy or made them uncomfortable, this is a good time to eliminate them from their sexual repertoire. Healthy sexuality includes only those sexual acts that are mutually consensual. A period of celibacy allows time for reflection on the entire sexual relationship.

Human beings commonly desire intimacy in their committed relationships. But for the sex addict, because he or she frequently divorces emotion from sex, intensity is often substituted for intimacy. Healthy sexual relationships may indeed have times of great intensity. But a defined period of celibacy allows couples to carefully examine their sexual relationship and choose to have it defined by true intimacy rather than frequency and intensity.

Celibacy contracts may be started at the beginning of recovery. It is best to enter into these contracts under a therapist's supervision. And since such contracts frequently take place prior to a formal disclosure, the partner does not know whether or not the sex addict partner has been sexual with other persons. Regardless of whether the acting-out behavior was that of the husband or the wife, this is a good time for both to have tests for sexually transmitted diseases. For the sake of health, the partner must assume there is a possibility he or she has been exposed to STDs.

For some couples, a celibacy contract is entered into while they are working toward disclosure. This is a period when the partner typically experiences a mixture of feelings as she or he waits for the addict to give details about acting-out behaviors. The partner is relieved from any pressure to perform sexually at a time when he or she feels most vulnerable. This is also a time when the addict can focus on exploring all of his or her acting-out behaviors in preparation for the disclosure and not use sex to medicate any feelings this may have stirred up.

Celibacy Contract Structure and Terms

The following is the basic celibacy contract used at Hope & Freedom Counseling Services. Although this contract addresses most of the addict's behaviors, conditions specific to a particular relationship can be added.

CELIBACY CONTRACT FOR COUPLES

The Sex Addict's Commitment

As part of my ongoing recovery, I have admitted to myself
that I have become powerless over my sexual behavior.
In order to maximize my recovery, I agree to abide by the
conditions of this contract. I will refrain from engaging in:

- Sexual behavior of any kind. (This includes sexual
or sensual touch and open-mouth kisses.)

- Appearing nude or semiclothed (exhibitionism).

- Masturbation.

- All seductive behavior.

- Pornography of any kind and all sexually suggestive media.

- All sexual conversations or suggestive innuendos.

- Any and all other sexual behavior.

- I will report sexual fantasizing to my therapist,
my weekly twelve-step group, my sponsor, and
my weekly therapy group with the desire of gaining
support as I maintain this celibacy period.

The purpose of this contract is to help remove sexually
dependent behaviors, cope with fantasy, and link me back
to healthy sexuality. Adherence to this contract may
result in recall of many childhood memories. Anxiety
will probably increase, as I will be unable to use my
sexual behavior as a coping mechanism. My groups,
my therapist, and my sponsor need to be aware of my
celibacy contract so that they can be of support to me.

Spouse's/Partner's Commitment

As the spouse/partner of a man/woman who is in treatment for problematic sexual behavior, I realize I have a responsibility to support my partner in this celibacy contract. For the duration of the contract period, I pledge to do the following:

• Not engage in sexual behavior of any kind.

• Not engage in any seductive behavior with my partner.

• Do all within my power to support my partner's desire to remain celibate for the duration of this contract period.

• Report any attempts made by my partner to be sexual or seductive.

• • •

This contract is in effect for _____ days starting today, _____. (Checkup therapy sessions will be scheduled with the couple every thirty days during the contract period.)

This contract is scheduled to be reviewed on _____. However, the contract will only end when mutually agreed upon by the couple and the therapist *during a therapy session*. (Prior to the expiration of this contract, the therapist will prepare the couple for resuming their sexual relationship with each other.)

CLIENT SIGNATURE   DATE

SPOUSE/PARTNER SIGNATURE   DATE

THERAPIST SIGNATURE   DATE

A celibacy contract requires cooperation from both partners. Not only must the addict make a commitment to not being sexual, but the partner also needs to be willing to give up sex for a defined period of time. This may be frightening to the partner of an addict because of her fear the sex addict will search for sexual release somewhere else if he does not have a sexual outlet at home. But the partner needs to remain firm and not resort to seductive behavior, which some individuals do when they wonder if their partner still finds them attractive. It is a painful period that must be endured if a couple chooses to enter a celibacy contract.

The couple is prepared for the period of celibacy through education as to its benefits and the fact that the celibacy is temporary. It is equally important that consideration be given as to how to end the celibacy contract. The couple is told that the contract can only come to an end during a therapy session when it is unanimously agreed to by the husband, the wife, and the therapist. If the wife or husband is seeing a different therapist, both therapists need to be in agreement for the contract to end.

In restarting the sexual relationship, there is value in encouraging the couple to continue to abstain from sexual intercourse for the first several sexual encounters. The emphasis should be on getting to know each other better and on providing pleasure for each other. The elimination of any expectation of intercourse will allow the couple to grow in their appreciation of each other and eliminate any performance anxiety that may accompany the end of the celibacy period.

THE PARTNER'S JOURNEY TOWARD RECOVERY: STOP THE CRAZY TRAIN!

Author's note: The following chapters contain therapeutic matter that is directly addressed to both the sex addict and his or her partner, in addition to general information about sex addiction.

Recovery Begins with Awareness

The process of recovery begins with the awareness that there is a problem. The sex addict may tell his or her partner that things are all in the partner's mind or that he or she is crazy, or even that he or she should be ashamed of his or her suspicion—it may even be suggested that the partner's suspicions are crazy. This is nonsense.

Partners: It is time to stop the crazy train! Your recovery will allow you to regain your stability. When you first became apprehensive about your partner's behavior, all you may have known was that things did not add up. Your partner would say that he or she was working late, and at first you believed the excuse. But when your suspicions grew and you mentioned your concerns, your partner dismissed you by saying that you were imagining things or that it was "all in your head." He or she may have gotten angry and caused a big scene. Your partner may even have shamed you for your feelings or made fun of you. What makes this especially troubling is that you may have even held the evidence in your hand, only to hear your partner say you are just imagining things. No wonder you may feel crazy.

Partners of sex addicts usually have an intuition that something is wrong. Sometimes there is no reason to be suspicious. Sometimes suspicions result from an overactive imagination or the projection of one's fear that the current partner is as unfaithful as a previous partner was, or perhaps it is the result of watching too many TV and movie melodramas. Sometimes, though, suspicions are well-founded. I have talked to numerous individuals who said that their partner (the sex addict) was so believable that he or she succeeded in convincing them that they were imagining a problem. One result of being told for years that they are just imagining things is that some people learn to dismiss their inner voice that tells them something is truly wrong.

What do you know? A useful starting point is to focus on what you know for certain. In making sense out of your concerns, write down what you know with certainty. It doesn't matter if your partner has acknowledged whether those things are true or not. What matters here is that you know that they are true.

What do you suspect? Next, make a list of the things that you suspect. For this list you will include those things that just do not add up. For example, your partner may have unaccounted-for time and not have a good explanation for what was happening during that time. Or your partner may have started some behavior that is in marked contrast to what has been the norm. For example, you may have noticed that your partner is a lot more concerned about appearance than in the past. You notice more care in clothing selection or more time spent on grooming.

Maybe you have noticed that your partner seems to be preoccupied with something and, based on past behavior, you don't think the concern is about his job. Once again, it doesn't matter if your partner agrees with the list or not. This list is for you. I would encourage you to keep the contents of this list to yourself. The purpose of the list is to help you think through things that are going on so that you can return to a place of sanity. The place to begin is to focus on what is known. Start with the following questions and ask if any of them fit your partner. However, don't jump to conclusions. There are legitimate reasons why a person may have one or several of these behaviors.

Behaviors Surrounding the Suspected Sex Addict's Work

- Has your partner stayed after work a lot and not been able to adequately explain why?

- Has your partner had to work on the weekends recently, although that has not been required in the past?

- When staying at work late, is your partner not available by phone?

- Has the number of your partner's business trips increased without explanation?

- When you offer to accompany him or her on a business trip, does your partner find reasons why that would not be a good idea?

- Does your partner describe a relationship with a coworker as being "just friends"?

Behaviors Surrounding Appearance

- Has your partner started dressing better?

- Has your partner started working out or losing weight or getting his or her hair colored, started using cologne or perfume, or started focusing more attention on personal appearance?

- Does your partner keep an extra change of clothes in the car or at work without a plausible explanation?

- Has your spouse left the house wearing one outfit and come home dressed differently?

- Does your partner smell fresh and clean (as if he or she just showered or used cologne or perfume) at the end of the day?

- Has your partner inexplicably laundered clothes or dropped off a single piece of clothing at the dry cleaner's?

Behaviors Surrounding Cell Phone and Other Mobile Information Technology Use

- Does your partner often not answer his or her cell phone when you call?

- Does your partner sometimes not answer his or her cell phone when with you? (Perhaps your partner looks at the screen and then says the call is not important.)

- Does your partner try to end cell phone calls hurriedly when you are around?

- Has your partner started sending and receiving text messages when that has not been part of his or her pattern of communication?

- Does your partner get phone calls that have to be taken in private? (Certainly there are appropriate times when privacy is necessary, but an unexplained need for privacy causes suspicion.)

- Has your partner purchased a calling card for no apparent reason?

- Have you discovered that your partner has purchased an additional cell phone that is kept in a secret place or is left at work?

- When your phone rings at home, do the persons calling often hang up when you answer?

- When your partner answers the phone, does he or she frequently say, "You have the wrong number," and then hang up?

- Does your partner erase text messages or the record of calls made or received?

- Has your partner acquired a smartphone, tablet computer, or some other device that allows him or her to be in constant email contact without a plausible explanation for why he or she needs the device?

Behaviors Surrounding Your Communication

- Does it seem that you and your partner are having arguments more frequently, sometimes followed by his or her leaving the premises?

- Has your partner started questioning your daily schedule more frequently?

- Have you caught your partner in lies both large and small?

Behaviors Surrounding Your Partner's Use of Time

- Is your partner frequently unavailable for family outings and activities?

- Are there periods of time when your spouse cannot account for his or her whereabouts?

- Does your partner get defensive if you ask about his or her schedule or erratic behavior?

- Does your partner get angry if you ask where he or she has been?

Behaviors Surrounding Money

- Has your partner started using cash for daily purchases rather than using credit cards or checks?

- Are there numerous cash withdrawals (from banks or ATMs) that your partner cannot adequately explain?

- Has gasoline usage suddenly increased more than normal?

- Are there receipts for gasoline purchases at stations that are well outside of your partner's normal traffic pattern?

- Does your partner get irritated when you ask questions about the family finances?

- Have you discovered a secret account, credit card, or stash of money?

- Does your partner have unexplained credit card charges?

- Does your partner take company expense reimbursements in cash?

- Has your partner recently moved significant sums of money from an account but not been able to give you a good reason for the move?

- Has your partner made decisions with your family finances that seem reckless or irresponsible, like closing accounts, removing your name from accounts, taking out loans, or changing the way retirement accounts are set up?

Behaviors Surrounding Computer Use

- Does your spouse use suggestive screen names when he or she gets on the Internet?

- If you enter the room and your partner is working on the computer, does your partner hurriedly close a program or make some quick movement to keep you from seeing what is on the screen?

- Have you noticed an increase in pornographic "spam" email on your home computer?

- Has the history in your Internet browser been erased?

- Have you found pornographic images on your home computer?

- Has your spouse purchased a webcam, scanner, or digital camera for what seems like a contrived reason, or tried to convince you of the need to make such a purchase?

- Does your partner get up in the middle of the night, saying he or she cannot sleep, then start working on the computer?

- Have you previously caught him or her looking at pornography or being involved in some other cybersex activity? Has your partner made promises to stop, but does the behavior continue?

Behaviors Surrounding Sex

- Has your partner's sexual appetite changed recently?

- Is your partner suddenly more interested in sex than in the past?

- Has your partner's sexual appetite diminished significantly?

- Has your partner started using new sexual moves or positions?

- Has your partner started to pressure you to do some things sexually with which you are not comfortable?

- Has your partner asked you to go to a sex-oriented or "adult" business when that has not been part of your past practice?

- Has your partner abruptly adopted a rigid, judgmental attitude about persons who engage in behavior that you would consider unacceptable? (This attitude may or may not concern some sexual behavior.)

The presence of any one or even of several of these things is not proof that there is a problem. You are in a discovery process, and the preceding questions simply serve to guide that process. If you are noticing things that seem unusual, there may or may not be anything to be concerned about.

However, as I have described, sex addicts can be crafty. While I do not recommend the procedure, some partners of addicts have hired private investigators to find out if their suspicions have foundation. Sometimes they learn that their partner has not been doing anything that would be considered inappropriate. Other times they find out that their partner's unexplained absences or financial expenditures were the result of something like taking dance lessons to surprise them, or that he or she has been involved in some other innocent behavior. But there are occasions when the investigator provides irrefutable proof that a partner has been acting out sexually. Such proof may be devastating. But it may also be affirming to know that the partner was not being unreasonably suspicious.

There are countless stories of individuals who have found a stash of pornographic photos on the family computer or the browser history shows that numerous pornography websites have been visited. Women have found receipts to sexual massage parlors or strip clubs, seen their partner sneak out of a neighbor's house in the middle of the day, or observed some other behavior that cannot easily be explained. Women, too, have acted out extensive sexual relationships over the Internet, and, in other cases, carried out extramarital affairs. Be certain not to let suspicious behavior cloud your thinking such that you make a leap and call suspicions fact. But if you do have proof your spouse has been involved in unacceptable sexual behavior, you are faced with a choice: What do you do with what you now know?

Confrontation and Intervention

What do you do once you know for certain that your partner is involved in sexual behavior that is outside of what has been agreed upon in your relationship? You can choose to ignore it. Perhaps that is what you have done in the past. Have you had proof of past indiscretions and dismissed them with the hope that they were onetime anomalies? Maybe you convinced yourself that if you didn't confront your partner with what you knew, things would get better. If you have practiced denial in the past, how has that worked for you? The fact that you are reading this book indicates that it did not have the desired results. Ignoring the problem will not make it go away. If your partner is an addict, your partner will not outgrow his or her addiction. The only remaining options are these:

- **Terminate the relationship.** Decide you have had enough and that your partner probably will not or cannot change. End the relationship and try to put the pieces of your life back together. Or:

- **Fight for your relationship.** Insist that your partner get immediate help to permanently stop all of the destructive acting-out behavior.

The second option is not the same as giving your partner a second chance. This option calls for you to determine that you are not going to continue living with a person who acts out sexually, and that there are no acceptable excuses for his or her past behavior. The fact that your partner is a sex addict does not relieve him or her of responsibility for the actions in the past or present. The recovering sex addict must take responsibility for what was done to you and your relationship. Most immediately, he or she must be willing to seek professional help.

When confronted with their behavior, some sex addicts continue to lie and deny that they have done anything sexually inappropriate. Others try to minimize their behavior by saying, "All men do it," or "It's just a guy thing," or "I just chatted with other men, I never met any in person," or even "I'm a sex addict, and I can't help it." They may respond with denials, anger, minimizing, rationalizing, or doing any number of other things to try to escape responsibility for their actions.

Numerous couples whom I work with would never have come to me if the partner had not finally gotten some hard evidence that his or her spouse was acting out sexually. There is such a focus on codependency in some recovery circles that virtually every behavior of the nonaddict may be seen as codependent. And there are those who would suggest that the partner should not try to get any evidence of sexual indiscretions based on the belief that such efforts are codependent. I beg to differ. I think to ignore what is going on around you and pretend nothing is going on when you have evidence to the contrary is an example of codependency.

If there is going to be hope for your relationship, then your partner must be faced with the evidence of his or her acting out. Until sex addicts can admit that they have a problem, they will not get help. Actual evidence can be enough to cause a person to make a break with the destructive behavior and finally get into recovery. Many of the couples I've worked with have a trusting relationship today because solid evidence of acting out was gathered by the partner of the sex addict, followed by both partners entering recovery.

Strive to Become an Expert

The next area of focus for you is to become an expert on the subject of sex addiction and recovery as well as on the partners of sex addicts. As if you had been diagnosed with a rare illness, you should approach your research of the subject of sex addiction with a voracious appetite. There are a number of websites that have a great deal of information about sex addiction and recovery. Learn all that you can. As you begin this learning process, one of the things I hope you get from your research is a sense of hope. Sex addiction is treatable, and relationships that are badly damaged by it can be restored. It is neither a quick nor an easy process. But relationships can be restored.

I hope you will read everything you can about sex addiction recovery. The next book you should read is *Your Sexually Addicted Spouse* by Barb Steffens and Marsha Means.[25] This book will give you a good understanding of the trauma that you have suffered.

Set Healthy Boundaries

This portion of the book is not meant to provide a comprehensive guide to setting healthy boundaries. Rather, it is intended to stimulate your consideration of the boundaries you want to set for yourself going forward. The first boundary to consider is whether it is acceptable to you to be in a relationship with a person who continues to act out sexually. If that is not acceptable, then you are on your way to setting one of your most important boundaries. When you set boundaries, you must determine how you are going to maintain those boundaries and what the consequences will be if they are violated.

If you determine that you are not going to be in a relationship with an individual who continues to act out sexually, then obviously you must tell your partner. You may prefer to do this in the presence of a friend or therapist for additional support. Avowing your boundaries is not the same as saying you are going to end your relationship with the sex addict. Sex addiction responds favorably to a combination of therapy and work in twelve-step fellowships.

When you are setting boundaries, work out ahead of time with your support system the full ramifications of establishing and enforcing those boundaries. This would preferably be with a therapist skilled at working with persons in relationships with sex addicts. In order for boundaries to be effective, there must be consequences in the event they are violated. It is essential that you consider what those consequences will be.

What are you prepared to do to back up the boundaries you have determined are necessary to protect yourself? When boundaries are violated without consequences, it is as if those boundaries do not exist. It also communicates that you will allow your boundaries to be disrespected, which is potentially worse than not setting boundaries to begin with. Are you willing to walk away from the relationship if your spouse does not get into recovery or otherwise does not respect the boundaries you have established? This is one of the most difficult decisions that you will make.

Contemplating the Possibility of Life on Your Own

For many people, it is frightening to consider separation. You are not looking for reasons to get out of your relationship. However, unless you take a stand that you will not remain with your partner if he or she continues to be sexual outside of your relationship, your partner may never stop acting out. Contemplating life on your own is not the same as making an empty threat. Rather, you are preparing to enforce your boundary not to be in a relationship unless love and sex are reserved exclusively for you. Are you emotionally ready to take this stand?

A helpful exercise is to keep a journal about various life situations and consider how you would handle them as a single person. If you have children, what will it be like raising them by yourself? How will you address all of the concerns—from child care to health insurance to transportation, not to mention housing and food—and do so by yourself, with whatever assistance you may have from family, friends, and others in your support system?

Healthy boundaries dictate that you have enough respect for yourself that you will not remain with a person who is unwilling to live in a monogamous relationship with you. The only way to back up that boundary is to be financially able to care for yourself in the event that the relationship ends. Are you financially ready to consider life on your own? Do you have the financial resources necessary to address the many concerns you will face if you are on your own? Do you have a job or career that will provide the ongoing financial support you need if you and your partner end your relationship?

If you do not have a job or a career, you need a plan. That may mean going back to work or further schooling to facilitate your independence. Regardless of your partner's situation, you may need to contemplate life without him or her—for your own sake, and if there are children involved, for theirs also. Do not misunderstand this to mean that you need to end your relationship. I am not advocating divorce or relationship termination without careful consideration and discussion. You need to decide what to do if the relationship ends and also be aware that there will be a number of legal concerns.

Protect Yourself Financially

It is imperative to protect yourself in the event your marriage or relationship ends. If you have confronted your partner over his or her sexual behavior and he or she is not willing to seek help, you need to make sure to look out for your interests and those of your children. Be alert for signs of suspicious activities regarding your assets, such as your partner moving money or closing accounts for no apparent reason. Has he or she opened additional accounts or made transfers that do not make sense? Do not sign anything regarding a financial transaction or a change in your business or a change in your mortgage if you suspect your partner is hiding things from you.

You may need an attorney immediately. This is not a prelude to divorce, but a preemptive move to protect your interests. You must not wait until assets have been moved and documentation hidden.

Such actions may seem like an overreaction. It is possible that your partner is not doing anything wrong with the family assets or hiding anything from you. But if you see any indications of this, it is in your best interest to protect yourself.

If and when you confront your partner with the ultimatum to seek treatment and recovery or end the marriage/relationship, don't be surprised if your partner says, "Fine, if that's the way you want it, then we can just live single." This response may be a test to see if you will back down. There is a chance that your partner may believe he or she wants to be single, and revel in the opportunity to act out without any accountability. That is a choice he or she will have to make. Before you capitulate or plead with your partner to stay, consider this: With no boundary to maintain, he or she may never seek help or enter recovery. What motivation does your partner have to change if he or she can enjoy the benefits of your relationship while continuing problematic sexual behavior at the same time?

Are you so desperate that you will stay with your partner under any circumstances? Or, to regain your self-respect, will you insist that the only way for you to stay in the relationship is for your partner to stop *all* of the extracurricular sexual activity and do concentrated work in recovery? If the choice comes down to it, is it better to have a spouse who cheats and will not tell the truth, or to have integrity and self-respect, knowing that you deserve an exclusive relationship? No one else can make these decisions for you. But once you make them, you will gain strength.

Partners frequently ask, "My spouse has begged me for a second chance. Should I grant it?" In some relationships, it is not a second chance that the addict asks for but a third, fourth, tenth, or hundredth chance. The answer must come from you. Do you believe your partner's sincerity enough to continue being with this person in spite of his or her transgressions? Is your partner engaged in a robust program of recovery that includes twelve-step meetings, working with a sponsor, and therapy? It is not enough to hear the words that they are going to change.

You have the right to expect to see a change in behavior, including your partner's participation in significant recovery activities. No matter the decision you make, you must take care of yourself. Consider engaging in individual therapy. Determine what behavior is acceptable for you and what is not. For those things that are unacceptable, set the boundary and hold firm.

Your boundaries do not determine your partner's behavior; they indicate what is important to you and how you choose to live. The courage to set and enforce healthy boundaries indicates your growing confidence as a person who does not have to settle for the leftover love of an unfaithful partner. You deserve more, and only you can stand up for yourself and say, "Unfaithfulness ends today!"

The Wounded You: Addressing Your Trauma

"My spouse is doing well in recovery. Why can't I get on with my life?" I hear this repeatedly from spouses and partners of sex addicts. The answer is elusive. There may be a number of factors at work. The heart of the difficulty is that partners have been traumatized by the discovery or disclosure of the sexual acting out.

Janelle's Story

Janelle has been in recovery for five years following the revelation that her husband, Tobey, was a sex addict. She worked hard and learned how to set healthy boundaries for herself. The first eighteen months after the discovery of her husband's problematic sexual behavior were very difficult. They continued to make progress and her husband got into recovery and was successful in stopping all acting-out behavior.

They sought the help of skilled therapists who understood sex addiction. Their recovery as a couple progressed well. Trust was slowly rebuilt to the point where after five years they had a much better relationship than before the discovery of his sex addiction.

Janelle believed she was completely healed of the trauma she suffered. It had been years since she worried if Tobey would act out again.

What has surprised Janelle is that a couple of times lately she has found herself getting profoundly sad as she thought about the early years of their marriage. Once she even dissolved into tears when a scene from a movie reminded her of the past. She immediately went back to her therapist and restarted her individual therapy.

After several sessions, her therapist concluded that Janelle had indeed largely healed from the trauma. The therapist also helped her to realize that while the trauma wound had healed, a tender scar remained. Sometimes she had some sadness about the past. That sadness was not an indicator that she was not doing well or had not done significant healing. Janelle realized that some of the impact of Tobey's acting out would continue to affect her in spite of the significant progress in recovery they had both experienced.

Following disclosure and a successful polygraph exam, sex addicts often feel relief. They finally have gotten their secrets out in the open. Perhaps they have a sense of satisfaction or even pride. They have finally told the truth. They may be looking for their partners to applaud their truth-telling and tell them how proud they are to be in the relationship. Partners may feel relief for knowing the truth, and also sadness and anger about what they learned. Many are traumatized, like survivors of war or persons who have witnessed a violent death or lived through a horrible natural disaster. Trauma may continue for years after the sex addict has achieved stable recovery and the couple system is otherwise healthy.

Stress or Trauma?

Everyone experiences stress and anxiety at one time or another. Stress occurs if you feel threatened or that you are in some sort of danger. Normal stress and anxiety responses may include loss of patience, agitation, anger, or withdrawal.

Trauma is stress on steroids. Trauma reactions may include waves of despair that result in uncontrollable sobbing. Traumatized persons may have such anger that they verbally attack, or such pain that they completely drop out of all activities for a time. Their emotional reactions are magnified and may be extreme. The results of several research studies indicate that following disclosure, partners of sex addicts often experience trauma. The study by Schneider, Corley, and Irons found that following disclosure the spouse felt hurt, betrayal, rejection, abandonment, devastation, loneliness, shame, isolation, humiliation, jealousy, and anger as well as loss of self-esteem.[26]

The most startling finding is that disclosure may propagate the features of post-traumatic stress disorder, or PTSD. In 2004, Coop-Gordon, Baucom, and Snyder found high levels of PTSD symptoms among partners within the first year following disclosure or discovery of an extramarital affair.[27] A study by Steffens and Rennie in 2006 found that 69.9 percent of participants met all but one criteria for diagnosis of PTSD using a tool known as the Post-Traumatic Stress Diagnostic Scale (PDS). They also found that 71.7 percent demonstrated a severe level of functional impairment in major areas of their lives as measured by the PDS.[28]

"I feel like I have just been kicked in the chest!" one man remarked after his partner's disclosure. "Why do I hurt so much?" said a wife after disclosure. Variations of this statement are made when spouses discover they are married to a sex addict. You may have feelings of sadness or anger. Perhaps the initial anger has been worked through, but there is still a terrible feeling in the pit of your stomach. What is going on? These are the effects of trauma.

Mental health professionals have come to expect that persons who have been at war or in a terrible accident, or who have witnessed a horrible atrocity, will suffer from aftereffects of trauma. During World War I, this was called "shell shock." Doctors noticed that patients might have early symptoms of irritability, tiredness, lack of concentration, or headaches. Some suffered from panic attacks and deserted. The doctors concluded that soldiers were suffering from the aftereffects of artillery shells exploding near them. It was wrongly theorized that the exploding shells created a vacuum that upset the cerebral-spinal fluid and upset the workings of the brain. This disorder has also been called "combat stress" and even "war neurosis." But we know that a person does not have to be in war to suffer from the same symptoms. People who have survived natural disasters, terrible accidents, or an act of great violence can also suffer in the same ways. The designations of shell shock and combat stress were replaced with post-traumatic stress disorder, or PTSD, during the 1980s.

PTSD is a neurological injury and not a mental illness. PTSD is a *natural* reaction to some *unnatural* situation. Historically, a criterion for diagnosing PTSD was the existence of a single major life-threatening event. Today there is growing recognition that PTSD may be caused by an accumulation of smaller events that, by themselves, are not life threatening. However, much of the mental health community still looks for a single life-threatening event to aid in the diagnosis of PTSD.

Other symptoms of PTSD may include flashbacks of traumatizing events, feelings of intense fear or helplessness, decreased interest or participation in important activities, or perhaps an inability to recall an important aspect of the trauma. Some persons suffering from PTSD report feelings of detachment or an inability to express loving feelings for their partner. Outbursts of anger, difficulty concentrating, changes in appetite, and sleep disturbances are also common. Some develop an exaggerated startle response, and others may become hypervigilant.

Does this relate to you? Have you been traumatized by revelations that your partner is a sex addict? You may have had multiple other traumatic experiences through the years that have added to the total weight of the trauma impacting you.

There are effective treatments for PTSD. A well-researched, nonmedical psychotherapeutic technique that targets PTSD is Eye Movement Desensitization and Reprocessing, or EMDR. This therapy helps process the troublesome memories and events to relieve PTSD.[29] In addition to EMDR, individual and group therapy using cognitive-behavioral techniques can help treat PTSD. Sometimes psychotropic drugs may also be helpful in treating PTSD. These are useful as long as the client is able to come to terms with the traumatic events. The most important first step is to see a therapist who is skilled in working with the partners of sex addicts and to have an assessment and evaluation.

Following disclosure, sex addicts must learn how to properly respond while the wounded partner works through his or her particular trauma. Through therapy, the recovering sex addict will be taught to validate the partner during the potentially lengthy time during which he or she is dealing with the trauma. The partner needs to be allowed to express anger and process the full range of feelings in order for healing to occur.

The discovery of your partner's acting out has had a significant traumatic impact on you. It is not realistic to expect a quick resolution to that trauma. The healing from your pain is a lengthy process. If you have experienced previous sexual or physical or emotional abuse in addition to your spouse's betrayal, you may need more extensive therapy to deal with those underlying issues.

The greater the trauma endured, the greater the need for you to be active in twelve-step recovery fellowships that support partners of sex addicts. Therapy and twelve-step meeting attendance are crucial to healing. The support network you build in these meetings will help to sustain you between therapy sessions and help make sense out of the insanity of addiction. While it is true that the addiction is the addict's, you have been deeply injured by it and need to give attention to your own healing. Treat yourself with kindness and seek your own recovery, whether or not your spouse is in recovery.

What About Forgiveness?

When does forgiveness come? Should it come? Sex addicts are eager to be forgiven. And some partners of sex addicts want to rush this process. This is especially the case where someone has a deep religious faith and believes forgiveness must immediately follow disclosure.

If your spouse commits him- or herself to recovery as a lifestyle, remains sexually sober, and treats you with gentleness and respect, forgiveness can come in time. Without you forcing it, as the relationship is restored, forgiveness will be a natural outgrowth of the work that both of you do in recovery. However, if you rush the forgiveness process, you may significantly slow the healing process for yourself and for you and your partner as a couple. I have had partners declare immediately after hearing a disclosure, "I forgive you. We will never speak of these things again." That may sound wonderful to a sex addict, but it is not helpful to a wounded partner or the health of the couple.

One of the myths about forgiveness is that in order to forgive, one must also forget. That is not true. You will likely never forget the things your partner has done that have harmed you. And he or she had better not forget how those things have wounded you. Remembering the past and taking action to see that those past behaviors are not repeated are necessary ingredients of recovery.

In order to heal from the past, you need to continue to talk about it, ask questions about it, and bring up things that concern you about the past. Premature forgiveness or cutting yourself off or allowing your partner to cut you off from being able to ask whatever questions you need to about the past is analogous to placing a bandage on an open but dirty wound. True, you cannot see the wound and may hope that it is getting better. But it will just get infected and the pain will fester.

Allow yourself to continue talking about the past and ask questions about the past for as long as you want. As you heal, if your partner can emotionally stay available to you through this process, you will gradually stop needing to bring up the past. If he or she is continuing to participate faithfully in recovery and does not get angry with you for bringing up feelings about his or her past behavior, you will heal. And with the healing, you will lose the desire to focus on the past.

If you come to the place of forgiving your spouse, do you declare that you have granted forgiveness? The test of forgiveness is not saying the words "I forgive you." You know from the sex addict's previous promises that "it will never happen again" that words, however earnestly intended, by themselves don't change feelings or behavior. It is possible to say those words but for forgiveness not to have taken place—because you simply are not ready to forgive. In the same way, you can forgive without declaring openly that you have forgiven your sex-addicted spouse.

It may be that you never actually speak the words "I forgive you" to your spouse. For some sex addicts, hearing those words may signal to them that they do not need to continue going to twelve-step meetings or doing other recovery activities. The addict may feel that since you have forgiven him or her, there is no need to continue the recovery journey. And he or she would be mistaken.

CHAPTER 13

PARTNER'S SURVIVAL KIT—
POST-DISCLOSURE

While every partner's response to a disclosure is individualized, the common thread is that disclosures almost always bring pain. Some may wonder, why then go through a disclosure? Why willingly put oneself in a position to be wounded? The answer is that you have a right to know the person you are in a primary/marital relationship with. And you have a right to know how their behavior has impacted your life. If there is to be a future together, it must be based on honesty—even though you know you will not like the things that you learn.

Hopefully, you will be fortunate enough to have a full, clinical disclosure. And if it is truly a full disclosure that has been verified with the use of polygraph, then you will most likely have received a lot of additional information about your partner's acting out. But you owe it to yourself to end the torment of imagining what your partner has done.

If you receive the disclosure as part of an inpatient or intensive outpatient treatment program, then you will also do some work after the disclosure to help you cope with the new information and the trauma it evokes. You may even have a sense of hopefulness following some of the post-disclosure work. Often partners have a sense of relief that the disclosure is over and they no longer have to wonder what has happened in the past.

Whether the disclosure comes as part of a larger treatment program or it is scheduled with your therapist as one of a number of weekly therapy sessions, you need to prepare for a significant emotional upheaval in the days and weeks following the disclosure. It is natural to feel a mixture of anger, sadness, hopefulness, rage, and relief, as well as many other emotions. You may have a time when you feel numb and cannot seem to function. You may also experience a number of physical symptoms ranging from pain in your muscles to shortness of breath, chest pains, sleeplessness, and loss of appetite. There may be projects that you start but cannot finish. You may find that you do not want to do much of anything. These symptoms may be part of your trauma reaction.

Trauma Triggers

As I described in the last chapter, the process of disclosure is often traumatizing. As a result, after you go through a disclosure, it is prudent for you to anticipate that some degree of trauma will be triggered. Some of these triggers can be anticipated. But others may come without warning and at the most inopportune times. If your partner acted out in your home, anticipate that just going home again will bring a whole raft of emotions. Some women have reported that this experience was made easier by asking a close female friend to meet them at their home and walk through it with them. Going from room to room and talking out loud about their feelings helps them to process some of the initial trauma. Others choose to walk through their home with their partner and talk about their feelings as they move from place to place.

Other common trauma triggers are hearing names of people your partner acted out with or watching a television program or movie that has sexual content. Normal conversations with friends or coworkers can be traumatizing if the subject matter touches, even briefly, on some behavior that your partner confessed to you. Any of the persons, places, or things associated with your partner's sexual acting out can trigger a traumatic reaction. It is also traumatizing to remember listening to your partner speak of his or her acting out. Time that you spend by yourself can be some of the most difficult. Even if you are in the presence of others through the day, when you try to sleep, you may find that sleep comes slowly and fitfully.

Make a list of all of the trauma triggers that you can identify. This will be a beginning point because you may find that there are numerous other things in life that may activate your trauma. After compiling this list on a sheet of paper, to the right of each trigger record at least one thing you can do to counter that trigger. Depending on whether the trigger is associated with a person, a circumstance, or a given situation, your plan to address that trigger can be tailored to the immediate need. It is helpful to work with your therapist and twelve-step support system in compiling this list of trauma triggers and your planned response to each trigger.

The following is a list of things some partners use when they encounter trauma triggers:

• Take deep breaths.

• Call a supportive friend.

• Call your sponsor.

• Pray.

- Recite Scripture.
- Hum a song.
- Journal.
- Work a puzzle that requires concentration.
- Talk to your spouse/partner.
- Engage in a hobby.
- Volunteer for a cause you are passionate about.
- Exercise.
- Practice good self-care.
- Get a manicure or a facial.

Now add additional things you can do to address your triggers.

If your partner is in recovery and is at a place where he or she wants to be supportive of your healing process, consider sharing this list with him or her. If he or she is sensitive to your needs, he or she will be interested in knowing the things that make life more difficult for you. You can learn to navigate life through the minefield of your triggers.

Hopefully your partner will understand if you need to leave certain places that activate your trauma. Some couples have agreed on a prearranged signal they can use to indicate to each other that they would like to leave particular events. The signal given by the sex addict may indicate that he or she recognizes that the environment is not conducive to his or her recovery. Or when the wounded partner gives the signal, it is an indicator that the situation is bringing up old memories or is in some other way triggering past trauma.

Assembling Your Survival Kit

Prior to the disclosure, you can prepare for what you are going to face. One of the best ways to prepare is to assemble a partner's survival kit. Below is a list of items that you can place in this kit. As you begin putting your kit together, be creative in adding additional items that you think might be helpful.

- Journal (use this multiple times each day to record your feelings and thoughts).
- *Stop Sex Addiction: Real Hope, True Freedom for Sex Addicts and Partners.*
- *Your Sexually Addicted Spouse: How Partners Can Cope and Heal.*[30]
- Phone numbers of close friends.
- Phone number of therapist.
- List of local meetings of twelve-step groups for partners of sex addicts like ISA, COSA, and S-Anon.
- List of activities that are self-soothing and/or make you feel pampered (like taking a walk in a park, taking a hot bath, getting a manicure/pedicure, etc.).
- Affirmations (make a long list of positive things about yourself that you know to be true). Do not hold back in an effort to be modest or humble.
- Your favorite photograph of yourself (this will be helpful as you remind yourself that you have value and worth and that your partner's acting out is not your fault).
- Scripture and/or a devotional or meditation book.
- Phone number of your spiritual adviser (e.g., minister, priest, rabbi).
- Some women have found things like a favorite fragrance or some scent used for aromatherapy helpful to get them in touch with their senses.
- Exercise clothes (vigorous physical exercise has significant mental health benefits).
- If you play a musical instrument, you may find it helpful as you process your emotions.
- Music CDs (a variety of your favorite music).

- A favorite blanket, wrap, or shawl.

- A stuffed animal that you can hold and squeeze.

- Any other items that might bring you comfort.

Assemble your kit in anticipation of receiving the disclosure. Not only are the items in this kit helpful for dealing with trauma, but the exercise of gathering the items will provide comfort as well as an activity to focus on, lessening the tendency to ruminate about the disclosure.

Beyond Your Kit

Following disclosure you may not want to be around anyone. But one of the unhealthiest things you can do is to isolate yourself. Break the impulse to isolate by spending time with a trusted friend. Call your therapist. Attend a twelve-step meeting. If you have already engaged a sponsor, this would be the ideal time to reach out to this person.

Your focus needs to be on self-care. What makes you feel good? What are the things that give you energy? It may seem selfish to you to think about yourself. But this is a time for some very healthy selfishness.

Nothing in your life has prepared you for the trauma of discovering that your partner is a sex addict and listening to a clinical disclosure of his or her sexual acting out. This is a time for being especially kind and gentle with yourself. Do not expect that you can go on with all of your normal responsibilities. Some find it helpful to take a week off from work or away from their usual activities immediately following the disclosure. Others find it therapeutic to maintain their regular schedule and activities as they mentally sort through what they have learned. Do not worry about anything or anyone else. If you have childcare responsibilities, enlist your spouse or a trusted friend to help out so that you can have time to contemplate what you have learned during the disclosure. Do not be afraid to ask for what you need. Take care of yourself. You deserve it!

CHAPTER 14

SURVEY RESULTS: THINGS THAT HELPED PARTNERS HEAL

In preparation for a video series for partners (www.imustheal.com), a survey was emailed asking for input from the partners of sex addicts. This survey was sent to current clients and also to over 1,200 others who have signed up at www.hopeandfreedom.com to receive our periodic newsletter. A total of 103 responses were received.

The purpose of the survey was to hear from a larger group of partners about their experiences in recovery. They were asked a number of general questions about recovery and some specific questions about healing and trust. Chapter 17 discusses the survey results concerning the restoration of trust in the sexual addict. Additional comments from the respondents can be found in Chapter 19.

AGE OF RESPONDENTS

One of the first surprises of the survey was the age of the respondents. Survey participants were older than anticipated. The single largest age group was 50–59, and the second largest was the 40–49 group. In fact, those two groups accounted for about two-thirds of the responses (see Figure 1).

FIGURE 1

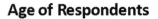

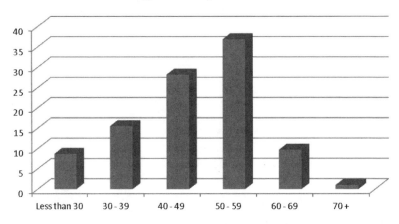

Age of Respondents

RELATIONSHIP TO SEX ADDICT

The survey asked about the relationship of the respondent to the sex addict. Of the 103 respondents, ninety-two were married and three were in committed relationships with sex addicts. But one of the realities of sex addiction is that four were already divorced, three indicated they were married but separated, and three more said they were in the process of getting a divorce (see Figure 2).

FIGURE 2

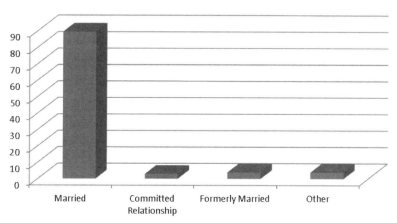

Relationship to Sex Addict

HOW LONG PARTNERS HAD KNOWN

Another unexpected result of the survey was how long the partners knew about the sexual acting out. Almost half of the respondents knew about their partner's acting out for at least three years, and more than fifteen percent had been aware of their partner's behavior for more than ten years (see Figure 3).

FIGURE 3

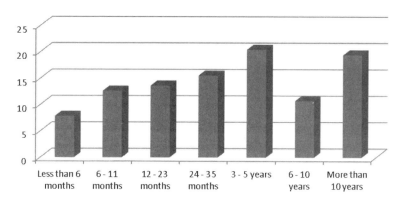

How Long Have You Known of Partner's Addiction?

HOW PARTNERS FOUND OUT

A little over 60 percent of respondents discovered their partner's acting out themselves. Of the couples I have worked with, the percentage of partners discovering acting-out behavior on their own is significantly higher. Conversely, relatively few sex addicts whom I treat have volunteered the information to their partner before their partner discovered it on his or her own. However, in this survey over 18 percent of participants said their partner volunteered information about their acting out before they were discovered. Five percent of those surveyed found out about their partner's acting out because someone else told them (see Figure 4).

The remaining 16.5 percent of survey participants found out about their partner's acting out in other ways. For example, two persons found out because their partners were arrested. One of these said she first found out when the FBI showed up at her door. Eight respondents either made a partial discovery or had suspicions and confronted their partner, and at that point the sex addict revealed more behaviors. One of the participants said she found out when her husband was diagnosed with AIDS. Two said they contracted STDs from their husbands. One of these said she was diagnosed with syphilis and then her husband confessed to acting out. Four respondents said they found out in a counseling session.

FIGURE 4

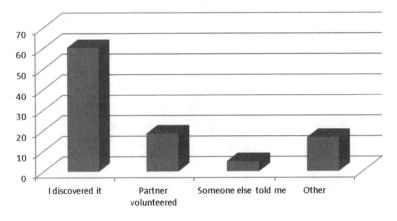

How They Found Out

WHERE PARTNERS IDENTIFIED THEMSELVES ON THE JOURNEY TOWARD HEALING

Respondents were asked where they were on the journey toward healing. Based on their own individual criteria, the respondents indicated whether their partner had made "significant," "some," or "no" progress. It was surprising how much progress had been reported by partners. Over 52 percent said they had made significant progress in healing. Nearly 41 percent said they had made some progress in healing. Fewer than 7 percent said they had not yet begun to heal (see Figure 5).

FIGURE 5

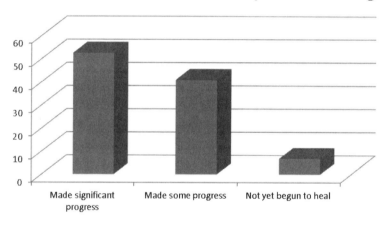

Where Are You on the Journey Toward Healing?

WHAT HELPED THE HEALING PROCESS AND WHAT DID NOT?

The survey allowed for respondents to indicate what was most beneficial to helping them heal and what was least beneficial. First, we will look at the things that were least beneficial. The responses are grouped according to where the partners were in their healing process. For this chapter and also for the survey results that are in Chapters 17 and 19, I have purposely deleted references to the work we do in our practice. My purpose in these chapters is not to promote our work but to find those more universal things that partners have found helpful to their healing, as well as those that were not helpful. References to our Three-Day Intensive program are grouped with other intensive outpatient programs. I have also left out references to processes that are unique to our treatment program.

A number of the treatment components and processes we use, such as disclosure, polygraph exams, and weekly check-ins, are used by many treatment providers. It is of interest that some of the things that are very helpful to some partners are not helpful to others. For example, there are several who talk about how helpful twelve-step meetings for partners are for their recovery. But there are others who are very vocal that those programs have not helped them. Some speak about how helpful therapy has been, yet others indicate they have been harmed by poor therapy.

You are unique. So is every individual. Some of what is offered by other partners will not be helpful to you. But there is also great wisdom that has been shared by the partners who completed the survey. Their insights can be helpful to your own journey of recovery. Of course, of particular note are the responses of those partners who have made significant progress in healing. By focusing on what has helped them, hopefully you will be able to make greater progress in your own healing.

The responses are grouped as much as possible. The respondents to this survey were most generous with their answers, and many of the answers were several paragraphs long. Most of the responses quoted here were shortened significantly in the interest of being able to include as many as possible in this book.

A Note to Male Sex Addicts

I do not think it is possible for male sex addicts to ever fully appreciate the depth of the pain inflicted on their partners. Many little girls dream about what life will be like when they grow up. If they are dreaming about getting married, they have wonderfully romantic fantasies about the person they will marry and how he will support them emotionally.

What is not part of any of their dreams is that they would fall in love with a sex addict who would hurt and abuse them. Your partner never dreamed that you would be unfaithful to her. She has trusted you with her life and health, only to have her trust shattered. You may not like the use of the word *abuse* to describe what you have done to your partner. But your sexual acting out has been abusive to her. The pain that you have inflicted may be deeper than if you had physically beaten her up. The damage you have inflicted with your penis is worse than any harm you could cause with your fists.

So how do you feel about yourself? Are you proud of what you have done to her? I know my words are strong. They are intended to have a sobering impact on you. Try to put yourself in her shoes. See if you can get even a glimmer of the pain that you have caused her.

Whatever previous traumas your partner has experienced will reemerge because of the trauma you have caused. Every person who has ever hurt her will coalesce into a monster that has your face, your voice, and your mannerisms. You become the one who is guilty of any abuse she has ever suffered. And you are the one who has inflicted all previous harm on her.

Is this fair? No, it is not. But that is the way trauma works. Of course, it is also not fair that you have so badly injured your partner. She may be able to smile and mask the pain. But never forget that at the core of her being, she has received a wound that may feel to her as if it is fatal. And for some women, the pain is not only mental or emotional, but it is also physical. Physical symptoms resulting from psychological trauma are well documented. She is not faking it or being melodramatic to get your attention. She may lose motivation for doing even some of the simplest things in life.

And on top of all else, she may feel trapped. As she looks toward the future, she may not be able to see anything that gives her hope. And frankly, some women *are* trapped, at least temporarily. Your partner may have given up on the pursuit of education or career in order to support you in your educational and career goals. She may have chosen to focus all her efforts on raising your children and providing a supportive home life for you. Now she wonders how she can move forward financially if you are not in her life.

You may have a chance—a slim one to be sure—to rebuild things with your partner. The only chance you have will come if you can take recovery seriously, stop all acting out forever, and then devote your attention to giving your partner all of the support that she needs for as long as she needs it so that she can heal.

If you focus on recovery and expect her to "just get over it," you may do well in recovery but you will fail in your relationship. If you try to rebuild trust but do not take on recovery as a lifestyle,[31] you will also fail in your relationship. These may seem to be harsh predictions, but they are based on my experience in working with many couples whose relationships have been rocked by sex addiction.

I have found that the difference between relationships that succeed and those that fail has little to do with the type or degree of the acting-out behaviors. I have seen relationships fail where acting out was limited to looking at pornography accompanied by compulsive masturbation. And I have seen relationships succeed where the acting-out behaviors have included acting out with multiple partners over many years, and some that included numerous illegal activities. The key ingredient is doing solid recovery work, stopping all acting out permanently, and committing to being part of the healing process with your partner.

With this in mind, I hope you will read the results of the next part of this survey with particular interest. The partners who completed the surveys have shared this information out of their pain and out of their hope. Their words contain wisdom that you may not find in any other book or from any therapist. They are the words that come from being in the trenches of sex addiction. Their words can guide you as you seek to rebuild the relationship with your partner. Ignore their wisdom and dismiss what they say at your own peril. Read. Absorb. Learn. Then put what you learn to work in your relationship.

Partners Who Have Not Yet Begun to Heal

Regardless of where the survey participants were in their journey of healing, we suspected that there were some things that they found helpful and other things that were not helpful. It is interesting to note that some items found by some partners to be unhelpful were found to be helpful by others. Beginning with the group who said they had not yet started to heal, numerous things were listed that have been barriers to their healing.

WHAT WAS LEAST BENEFICIAL TO HEALING?

- Husband has not taken responsibility for his actions.

- Psychotherapy.

- Keeping some proof of the past, such as emails. When I felt down, I went back to some of them. No good came out of this.

- Talking to my husband.

- TV and movies.

- Having a poor counselor.

- Husband blaming me.

- Husband minimizing his behavior.

- Husband's anger and resentment.

- Husband takes me for granted.

WHAT WAS MOST BENEFICIAL TO HEALING?

The partners who said they had not yet begun to heal nonetheless indicated that there were some things that they found helpful. They found the following items beneficial.

- Reading religious Scripture.

- Twelve-step meetings for partners of sex addicts.

- Husband working diligently on his program.

- Living separately for a time.

- Porn-blocking software.

- Husband willing to quit playing professional sports.

- Books about recovery.

- Taking long walks.

- Prayer.

- Crying.

- Therapy.

- Disclosure followed by a polygraph.

- Videos about recovery.

- Practicing good self-care.

Partners Who Have Made Some Progress in Healing

Nearly 41 percent of those surveyed said they had made some progress in healing. Again we asked what things were most helpful and which were least helpful. And once again we see that what was helpful for some was not helpful for others. First we look at what this group found to be least helpful.

WHAT WAS LEAST BENEFICIAL TO HEALING?

- Partner's continued acting out and deceit after discovery.

- Being labeled a "co-addict" (several respondents mentioned this).

- Codependent model of partner recovery (this was mentioned by several).

- The multitude of books that automatically label the partner as a codependent or co-addict and downplay any trauma the partner has experienced.

- His verbal commitment to change. ("I must see him actually walking the walk of recovery.") Words have little or no meaning.

- Twelve-step groups for partners.

- When I find out that my husband is still in contact with former partners.

- Pastors of several churches where I have sought help. They are good people but have no knowledge of the seriousness of the problem and the way to solve it and no awareness of the effect of the behavior on the spouse.

- Counselors without specific training in sex addiction.

- There is a tremendous need in Christianity to get the word out about sex addiction and how to heal it. All of the women in my twelve-step group are Christians and their husbands hold responsible positions in the church.

- Weekly check-in by my partner.

- Talking with well-meaning close church friends who do not understand sex addiction.

- False information in the media about sex addiction.

- Being blamed by sex addict's parents and friends.

- Being told by therapists I should "move on" and get over what my partner has done.

- Being told initially by my therapist not to talk about the addict.

- Geographical location. I live in Australia and there is not much recognition of the problem and there are not many sex addiction resources available here.

- Faked recovery by sex addict.

- Partner doesn't talk about his recovery.

- Partner's refusal to do a disclosure.

- I still have great difficulty during sex in believing that he really wants me.

- He obviously chose homosexual sex over sex with me from the beginning, so I long for some sort of reassurance that our marriage will ever give him the fulfillment he desires.

- My husband's inability to accept responsibility for his choices.

- Him blaming me and telling me that men who are happy at home don't stray.

- My husband showing me no remorse, no empathy, no sympathy, no love, no trust, no godly sorrow for deceiving me for over thirty years.

- He is unwilling to listen to my pain without him believing I am just doing this to blame or punish him.

- His belief that he can keep that part of his life secret from me.

- My husband telling our church family without my knowledge or permission. He does not realize that this is now my story also.

- I feel shame because I feel many blame me as the wife for his sexual acting out.

- I feel unwelcome, rejected, and abandoned, while he is welcomed back at church because he repented.

- Poor counseling with two therapists who didn't recognize how serious the addiction was. This ended with heavy expense and frustration.

- The close friendships that I have are all based on being able to talk about anything and everything. Because secrecy about his sex addiction is necessary, I cannot talk to my friends about my life with my husband. I cannot talk about my feelings about what I am going through. I really can't talk about anything to any of my friends or family. I have to keep secrets.

- Counselors telling me, "It's not that big of a deal. Women use prostitutes, too," or a different one saying, "If you knew what you know now, would you have married him? So why are you still here?" Another one saying, "You are too controlling," or another one telling me, "There's nothing I can do for you. Your husband won't be emotionally mature enough for a relationship for years," or "Even if you don't stay with him, he will make someone else a wonderful husband."

- Hard to be around happily married people.

- Twelve-step meetings for partners were helpful before disclosure but are too triggering now.

- Going to the wrong therapist who focused on the sex addict was not beneficial.

- Spouse's unwillingness to seek counseling to help heal. Lack of financial resources to attend counseling or purchase materials.

- I have observed that in the church there is an "old school" belief that if your spouse struggles with sex addiction, it's because the wife is not sexual enough with her husband.

- Trying to explain how I feel to my husband. Every time I do I get rejected and it causes more hurt and pain.

- Expecting change from him and believing his promises. It is better that I concentrate on me and take his words with a grain of salt.

- I did not make the best choice for a therapist, so therapy has not been as beneficial as it should have been. My therapist is very negative toward older sex addicts. I would like a more supportive point of view.

- Stopping my antidepressant medication for a few months.

- Being angry at God.

- My partner's lack of commitment to recovery.

- Recovering sex addicts and their partners do not get the same social support as those in other addictions.

- The media and others who think men just do things because they are men.

- Negative thinking, and not feeling my husband is making as much progress in recovery as I would like.

- Our therapist moved, so we have to find a new one.

- Listening to other women in my support group who are not having a good experience and whose husbands are not committed to recovery.

- Pastoral counseling and Christian counselors in general. I am a born-again Christian and these are good people but they don't have a clue what they are dealing with.
- My husband's long-standing pattern of withdrawal whenever anything upsetting or difficult comes up.
- Partner's defensiveness.
- Partner's depression.
- Lack of trust in my own judgment.

WHAT WAS MOST BENEFICIAL TO HEALING?

The respondents in this group also identified things that were most helpful in their healing. While some have mentioned how helpful therapy has been for them, it is also interesting to note that many of the things identified by this group had little or no cost involved. This is especially important for the many partners who simply cannot afford therapy no matter how much it might help. Here are the things this group found most helpful.

- Reading good recovery books.
- Attending twelve-step meetings for partners.
- Honesty from partner.
- Partner's commitment to twelve-step meetings and going to counseling.
- Disclosure.
- Working with a CSAT (Certified Sex Addiction Therapist).[32]
- Weekly self-reflection.
- Using the Recovery Points System.[33]
- Aftercare intensives with polygraph.
- During times of healing, my husband has been involved in a recovery program. Without me asking or urging, he voluntarily makes strides in recovery by attending meetings, talking to accountability partners, working on recovery materials, and attending church.

- Several respondents mentioned intensive outpatient programs they attended as being helpful.

- Ending the isolation. I no longer feel I am the only one hiding this terrible secret.

- Discussing issues with a very close friend.

- Several spoke about how helpful it was to have follow-up polygraph exams taken periodically in the months and years after a clinical disclosure to verify that their partner was in good recovery and that none of the problematic sexual behaviors had recurred.

- Talking in a group for partners of sex addicts.

- My husband's patience with my healing process.

- Journaling about my experiences.

- Various recovery websites, some of which are specifically for partners.

- Listening to music.

- Spending time with animals.

- Period of separation following my discovery of his acting out.

- After having no sexual contact in our marriage for over twenty years, we have begun to have sex again, so I don't feel as much like our marriage is a sham. He has begun to share some more concrete facts of what his behavior entailed.

- Realizing that this is a true illness.

- Having a therapist listen to me and acknowledge my pain.

- Taking care of my needs by attending twelve-step meetings and working the Twelve Steps. Finding friendships in the twelve-step program.

- Getting massages when needed, trying to eat healthier, resting, seeing my doctor regularly.

- Finding something I can have fun doing.

- My belief in God and meditating on His Word is one of the most helpful things to me.

- One older man from our church family is like a father to my husband and me, and has taken an interest in trying to help both of us. He knows the problems intimately and he does not take sides. He encourages my husband to be a godly man of integrity and to treat me as the Lord would have him do.

- Not getting my family involved in what is going on. To tell any of my family members would create chaos for me. It would involve embarrassment, judging, constant phone calling, and badgering. The less people who know, the better for me.

- My husband is finally recognizing and admitting his problem and taking steps toward repair.

- Counseling. My husband did not seek professional help for years for fear of what a charlatan sex therapist might do to our marriage. There was very little help available years ago. Finding the right professional help has been a godsend.

- Several mentioned taking medication for depression. Others mentioned medication for panic attacks early in recovery.

- Recognizing my codependent behaviors in all aspects of my life.

- Learning to stand up for myself more and never trusting blindly.

- Yoga.

- Learning that it was not my fault.

- I had my husband move out of the bedroom so I could create a safe space for myself.

- My husband has made a huge effort to stop the violence and rage toward me. *[Note from author: If he is violent toward you, do not try to reason with him. Get to safety immediately and call the police. Do this without regard to whether he is going to be mad at you. There is never any excuse for violence. This is also true for wounded spouses being violent with their sex addict partner.]*

• Detaching emotionally from my husband and his issues.

• Looking at my own history and exploring my own issues of fear, inadequacy, control, anger/rage, shame, entitlement, and reactions to pain.

• My decision to explore and embrace the concept of forgiveness for my own healing purposes.

• My husband's willingness to be 100 percent accountable to me and 100 percent committed to his recovery.

• I don't think we would be where we are today in recovery if our journey had not begun with a full disclosure and polygraph. Although it is difficult knowing it all, it also is beneficial knowing what I am dealing with.

• Him being totally open and honest with me. Him having a whole new attitude toward being a man and stepping up.

• Hearing other women's stories and having my feelings validated.

• The times my husband shut his mouth and let me rant about my anger.

Partners Who Have Made Significant Progress in Healing

Of perhaps greatest interest to those who are new in recovery are the experiences of partners who have made the most progress in healing. More than 52 percent of those responding to the survey reported that they have made significant progress in healing.

WHAT WAS LEAST BENEFICIAL TO HEALING?

Even with the significant progress that this group has made, there have been numerous things they have identified that were not helpful in their healing journey. Here is their list.

• Some women in the twelve-step group come back week after week telling the same story and staying stuck in the victim role. I found that to be a huge distraction in my healing. I prefer to be with people who move forward in their recovery journey and can help me do the same.

- Feeling like a leper in the community. Afraid of people finding out.

- Twelve-step meetings for partners (in person and by telephone).

- Reading self-help books about being the partner of a sex addict.

- Sharing/talking with friends who think sex addiction is about being a playboy.

- The co-addict label and being treated as a co-addict. This is a highly damaging method of treatment and it results in therapy-induced trauma. It must stop. (Eight partners in this group mentioned this item. Each of the comments was lengthy and expressed strong negative feelings about being labeled a co-addict simply because of being in a relationship with a sex addict.)

- Doctors telling me that I suffer from PTSD because then I become the victim. I had to stop listening to "the pros" and listen to me.

- I found that most spouses in twelve-step meetings typically end with "spouse bashing," and I don't need that.

- Traditional marital counseling by those who don't understand sex addiction.

- Dwelling on his actions and reliving the past.

- Bad advice and hurtful comments, especially from counselors and twelve-step leaders.

- Spending too much time on an online forum where there are wives of sex addicts and really no constructive moderating to help keep things focused on moving forward.

- Some recovery books, especially some from a Christian perspective.

- Reading books on how to be a better wife to keep my husband's attention.

- My husband's lies and his controlling the release of information.

- His pretending to work on recovery but continuing to act out and hiding it while telling me he was working on his recovery program as hard as he could.

- My husband telling me I will never heal and never get over this.

- My first counselor, whom I had known for two years, ending our counseling relationship because I kept saying I knew there was something else going on.

- Waiting for my husband to change.

- Blaming my husband for all of our marital problems.

- People giving advice when they don't understand sex addiction.

- Staying in the position of victim and martyr by repeating to others what he has done to me.

- Being with unsafe people and expecting them to understand in a healthy way.

- Staying with my spouse, who has never totally surrendered and only agreed to get minimal help when I threatened to leave.

- The church we were attending when he disclosed everything. I thank God for directing us immediately to another church where he could be totally honest and open and we both could get healing.

- Counseling in the beginning that concentrated on me and what I was doing wrong instead of dealing with the trauma I was experiencing.

- Making the mistake of telling people who know nothing about sex addiction.

- Expecting my husband to change for me.

- Expecting signs of caring, concern, and support for me from my husband.

- We live two hours away from our therapist and from any twelve-step meetings, so we have had to find ways around that.

- Having a controlling therapist who wouldn't give a specific disclosure date when I asked for it. The most traumatizing thing for me was waiting for the disclosure for six months.

- Trying to fix the addict. I can only control myself.

- Trying to get into his mind and understand what made him do such things.

- Condemning or trying to make him feel ashamed or guilty.

- Having sex with my husband too soon after the discovery of his addiction.

- Other people's opinions on how I should handle the situation. There are many opposing views trying to help.

- His taking too long to answer all my questions. Trickle truth.

- Not having an opportunity to discuss my feelings with our adult kids who live far away and not feeling they understand my deep pain.

- Attending family week when my husband was in an inpatient treatment facility and being labeled a co-addict. Also attending all-day grueling sessions there and then being thrust outside to a motel on my own each night.

- Hearing him say that he is a sex addict. It feels like it's an excuse to justify his behaviors.

- Having to continue working without the ability to take time off.

- My inability to set boundaries.

- Our inability to communicate and ask for what we need from each other.

- Our work schedules because we sometimes don't get to see each other.

- The constant triggers that I encounter on a daily basis.

- When he discounts me or pokes fun at my trauma triggers or is insensitive and disengages as a form of punishing me for questioning him.

WHAT WAS MOST BENEFICIAL TO HEALING?

This group, who reported having made significant progress in healing, identified many things that were most helpful to them in their journey.

- Reading recovery books.

- Finding a good, solid counselor who is trained in the treatment of sex addiction.

- Setting clear and solid boundaries to protect myself emotionally, physically, and spiritually.

- Twelve-step meetings for partners.

- Twelve-step meetings for couples in recovery.

- Openly talking about the addiction and recovery with my husband on a regular basis.

- Communication is the most important key that leads back to trust for us.

- Reaching out to others in need.

- Journaling.

- Therapy with a competent therapist.

- Going to a recovery group for codependency at church.

- Full disclosure and polygraph.

- Periodic follow-up polygraphs.

- You must be willing and able to leave the addict in the dust of your recovery if he or she cannot or will not move forward with you.

- I think that partners need to avoid identifying themselves as a victim. Acknowledge your pain, voice your pain, but don't live in your pain.

- Educating myself about sex addiction and about partner trauma.

- Faith and prayer.

- Praying together.

- Spiritual practices and spiritual leaders (partners who practice Christianity, Judaism, Buddhism, and Hinduism spoke of the help they receive from their faith).

- Realizing that I can't fix, change, or stop his behaviors.

- Camping with my dog.

- Having someone safe to talk to. Having my husband committed to the relationship and healing. Having a relationship with God, as He is the only one who will never fail us.

- Having good communication skills with each other.

- Weekly check-in by my partner.

- Talking with other women who are wives of sex addicts.

- Making a list of my losses and mourning each one and then moving on.

- Having a mentor for myself.

- Various recreational activities including kickboxing, biking, and running.

- Yoga.

- Woman Within weekends and e-circles.[34]

- Understanding that the only person I have control over is myself.

- Him taking responsibility for the distrust that is in our marriage.

- Attending workshops and seminars on recovery.

- Following the structured recovery program guided by a therapist specializing in sex addiction recovery.

- Working with a sponsor in a twelve-step program.

- Affirmations.

- Journaling.

- Time alone.

- Our pastor took the problem seriously without judging either of us.

- Doing some fun stuff alone, with friends, and with my partner once the healing had truly begun.
- Weekly date night.
- Continuing to talk about, plan for, and look forward to our future.
- Burning, selling, and getting rid of items associated with his adultery.
- Positive self-talk.

Of particular note is the number of women who have participated in telephone-based support groups facilitated by Marsha Means or one of the therapists and facilitators who work with her practice called A Circle of Joy. Ten of the respondents said these groups were instrumental in their healing. This was the single largest response for working with any therapist. These women also spoke of the resources on her website, www.acircleofjoy.com, as well as the book she and Dr. Barb Steffens wrote, *Your Sexually Addicted Spouse: How Partners Can Cope and Heal*.

As you consider the comments from others you have read in this chapter, I would suggest that you do not take a single comment or even several comments and make drastic changes in your recovery based only on them. There is a lot of experience and much wisdom here. Give some of these ideas and suggestions a try and then evaluate the results. As the wide range of these comments makes clear, different things work for different people. Only you can decide what is helpful for you.

If you make some changes in your recovery as a result of something you have read from these survey results and find that you have taken a step backward, then revert to your previous recovery direction. You may then consider some of the other things partners have suggested and see if they help you in your healing process. The best way to determine if something is a good fit for you is to try it on for size.

In Chapter 17 we will look at the survey results concerning the restoration of trust in relationships. But it is noteworthy that restoring trust is not a prerequisite for your individual healing. Twenty-two of the survey participants said they had no trust in their partner but have already experienced at least some healing. And nine of those surveyed said there is no trust in their partner but they have experienced significant healing.

However, generally those who have experienced at least some restoration of trust in their relationship have made more progress in their healing. Twenty-two respondents said they have only some trust in their partner yet have experienced significant healing. And twenty-one of the partners said they have experienced both a significant restoration of trust and significant healing.

![CHAPTER 15]

SLIPS AND RELAPSES IN RECOVERY

Freeman's Story

Freeman started his acting out long before the inception of the Internet. He recalls seeing some old detective magazines in a secondhand bookstore in the early 1960s. As a teenager, Freeman found his first soft pornographic "men's magazines" in a dumpster used to recycle newspapers and magazines. When he was a freshman in high school, a friend brought a nudist colony magazine to school. He traded his bicycle for the magazine, since it was the first time he had ever seen a photo of a nude woman. Freeman was captivated by what he saw and had to own the magazine.

As a young adult, he gathered every pornographic magazine he could find. Gradually, he started seeking out hard-core pornography but did not like having to go to the adult bookstores to get what he wanted. With the advent of the Internet, he was relieved that he could find what he wanted on the computer. By the time he got into recovery, Freeman was spending a significant portion of each day looking at pornography while at work. He was terrified when he heard that the technology department at his company had installed software that would allow them to determine which employees were violating the company computer policies.

After reading about sex addiction on the Internet, Freeman entered recovery. He attended twelve-step meetings, got a sponsor, and worked the steps. But gradually Freeman decreased his meeting attendance and stopped meeting with his sponsor. He reasoned that since he had gone several months without acting out, he was probably cured and did not need to continue his recovery activities.

Months later, Freeman had his first slip. He clicked on an Internet news story about the arrest of a celebrity. Two clicks later he was viewing hard-core pornography. This began a cycle of slipping, getting back into recovery, and then losing interest in going to meetings. The cycle continued to repeat. Freeman tried to stop his behavior many times, but each effort ended when he had a slip or entered a period of full relapse. He sought out the services of two therapists to help him deal with his problematic sexual behavior, but neither was experienced in treating sex addiction. He even had a religious experience during which he promised God that he would stop acting out. But none of these efforts provided him lasting relief from his addiction.

No one ever knew of his struggle, but the fear of being caught led him to seek a therapist who specialized in sex addiction to help him stop his problematic sexual behavior. With a solid reentry to recovery, he was finally able to establish long-term sexual sobriety. He now has over five years without acting out. As part of his recovery program, Freeman continues to attend three twelve-step meetings a week, is currently sponsoring several other men, and has one individual therapy session each month for added accountability.

Are Slips and Relapses Inevitable?

The answer to this question is no. While a large portion of the people entering recovery programs for all forms of addiction suffer setbacks or relapses, there are addicts in recovery who never slip or relapse. There should be an expectation of no slips or relapses. When individuals believe they are likely to slip, they risk setting themselves up for this to become a self-fulfilling prophecy.

Slips are significant events in recovery that call for immediate attention. Slips happen when the addict believes him- or herself to be "cured," is not prepared to deal with triggers to act out, and/or has slacked off in his or her recovery. Slips often result when addicts take risks by placing themselves in situations that are dangerous to their recovery, sometimes through exposure to circumstances and behaviors the sex addict has identified as problematic. Slips can be framed by the acronym SLIP: "Sobriety Lost Its Priority." A slip or a relapse is a wake-up call that the addict's attitude and actions must change.

Some sex addicts play games with themselves about defining what is acting out and what is just harmless behavior. They may be clear that they will never look at pornography again. But they see nothing wrong with looking at swimsuit magazines or websites, or viewing lingerie catalogs or other underwear ads. But solid recovery demands that a sex addict have a clear-eyed view of behaviors that can lead to relapse. For example, in the case of pornography, the definition of pornography for someone who is in solid recovery should include anything that is sought out to be tantalizing or provocative.

This may seem extreme. But to start back down a path with "near porn" (similar to "near beer") places the recovering addict on a path that leads to relapse. Starting any of these behaviors is the proverbial camel getting his nose under the edge of the tent. Once that happens, it usually isn't long before the entire camel is in the tent!

What Is the Difference Between a Slip and a Relapse?

A slip is a onetime event that happens unexpectedly and without planning. A relapse is a more substantial movement back into problematic sexual behavior. This may be a onetime event or a series of events. For example, a recovering addict who spends the night acting out with another person did not experience a slip but had a relapse. A recovering addict who has "slipped" and gone to an adult bookstore two weekends in a row has also experienced a relapse.

If one has a slip or a relapse, he or she must make immediate and perhaps drastic changes to prevent the problem behavior from recurring and worsening. If the individual does not change anything, he or she can expect the destructive behavior to continue to repeat as he or she once again becomes active in addiction. Sex addicts should take immediate steps to restart their recovery program in order to prevent further relapse.

People in recovery from any addiction may experience missteps along the way. In fact, there are some clinical professionals who teach that recovering persons should expect slips and perhaps relapses. Sex addicts try numerous things to stop their compulsive behavior before they get into solid recovery. Often, they have made attempts to control their sexual acting out before anyone else knew about their addiction.

The expectation that I set out for clients who are already in recovery is that they should not have a single slip after this point. Slips may be common in twelve-step circles, but that does not mean that a slip is inevitable. Sometimes there is debate in twelve-step recovery as to whether a behavior constitutes a slip or a relapse. There is an easy way of determining how a problem behavior is categorized. Remember "Dr. Pepper," or at least remember DRP. Three words can help you determine whether a behavior is a slip or a relapse:

Duration—How much time did the behavior consume? If a behavior is of a short duration, then it might be considered a slip. But the behavior that is of longer duration would be rightly categorized as a relapse.

Repetition—If a behavior is repeated, regardless of how short a time the individual behavior lasts, it qualifies as a relapse. A person may have a slip today. But if the behavior is repeated tomorrow, it is not another slip. Rather, a relapse started today.

Premeditation—If a behavior is premeditated, even if it is brief and not repeated, then it should be considered a relapse. If a behavior is planned to take place when your spouse is out of town, even if it is ultimately of short duration, the behavior should be called a relapse.

Why does it matter? The question on the mind of many sex addicts is whether they have to start over in counting their time in sexual sobriety. I believe the sobriety clock is reset with both slips and relapses. Any acting out, regardless of how brief, is still a breach of sexual sobriety.

For those who are set on minimizing their behavior by saying, "It was just a slip," caution is advised. Slips and relapses are both serious events that require assessing what in attitude and action is necessary to keep the behavior from happening again and to return to sexual sobriety. The importance of accurately defining a return to sexual acting-out behavior as a slip or a relapse lies in the type and intensity of the changes that need to be made moving forward. Does the event in question require entering or increasing therapy? Should intensive outpatient services be considered? Or is it time to finally go to an inpatient treatment facility?

Levels of Care (LOC) in Treatment

The process of getting back into recovery after a slip or relapse may be different for each person. It depends on whether the recovering addict experienced a slip or a relapse, as well as the behaviors involved. For a relapse, a critical consideration is the length of time the person was actively reengaged in their addiction.

"Levels of care" refers to the types of professional treatment options. Levels of care progress from least to most intensive. The appropriate level of care for each individual is that which is necessary based on the type of addictive behavior, its duration, and the resolve of the sex addict to make recovery a priority. The objective is to select the least intrusive level of care that adequately addresses the problem. For example, a slip involving "only" masturbation may call for using LOC (Level of Care) 2. However, a relapse with a return to other acting-out behaviors will call for LOC 3.

LEVEL OF CARE ONE (LOC 1)

LOC 1 is the basic level of care for clients who enter therapy. It involves weekly individual therapy sessions. Clients are expected to attend twelve-step meetings at least twice per week. After the client is stabilized and has gained a good foundation in recovery, he or she is encouraged to begin group therapy as an adjunct to individual therapy.

LEVEL OF CARE TWO (LOC 2)

This level of care involves an increase in twelve-step meetings and therapy. The person should begin or restart therapy. A combination of individual therapy and, after a person has established a good recovery foundation, participation in group therapy is recommended. Following a slip or a relapse, the addict should have therapy twice a week. Some may benefit from therapy even more frequently for several weeks. If the client is not in group therapy, he or she should get into a group as soon as possible. The increased therapy schedule should continue for three or more weeks, depending on how the client responds.

Level of Care Two requires attending three twelve-step meetings a week and, if time and schedule allow, increasing this number. For some it is helpful to increase twelve-step meeting attendance to one per day for ninety days, known as a "90/90." It may be difficult to find twelve-step meetings that deal with sex addiction every day of the week. However, this should not be seen as a reason to abandon doing a 90/90. Any twelve-step meeting may supplement a sex addict's regular meetings. When introducing him- or herself at meetings, the recovering sex addict can simply say, "I'm an addict from another fellowship." It is common for persons with various addictions to attend Alcoholic Anonymous or Narcotics Anonymous meetings to augment their other recovery meetings. Besides, quite a few addicts struggle with more than one form of addiction. There are also online and telephone-based meetings for twelve-step fellowships that a person can attend if he or she cannot find available meetings nearby.

With each level of care, the sex addict must contact his or her sponsor to ensure the sponsor is aware of any slip or relapse, and to indicate that he or she is open to direction on how to reestablish sexual sobriety. If the addict does not have a sponsor, he or she must get one immediately. The lack of a sponsor may be a significant contributing factor to a slip or relapse.

LEVEL OF CARE THREE (LOC 3)

LOC 3 calls for a brief intensive outpatient program focused on relapse recovery, such as the Three-Day Intensive program we offer at Hope & Freedom Counseling. These intensive programs are tailored specifically to the needs of the individual who has slipped or relapsed. Actions and attitudes that may have contributed to the slip or relapse are reviewed by the therapist, and the client is helped to reestablish sustainable recovery routines.

Three-Day Intensives, as we call them, are carefully coordinated with the client's home therapist, who also receives a copy of the client's discharge summary. Significant care is taken to ensure that the brief intensive treatment will complement the client's ongoing therapy. The Intensive culminates with the client being led through the construction and implementation of a Personal Recovery Plan. Most Intensives include an opportunity to take a polygraph exam to back up a disclosure of additional acting-out behavior.

As with LOC 2, there is also an increase in twelve-step meetings to a minimum of three meetings per week, and perhaps a 90/90. Attending these meetings should be seen as a priority for recovery. Unfortunately, there are some clients who view twelve-step meetings as optional since there is no cost associated with them. It is not surprising that clients slip or relapse when they drastically cut down on or stop attending recovery meetings.

LEVEL OF CARE FOUR (LOC 4)

LOC 4 involves longer intensive outpatient treatment for one to three weeks. There are excellent organizations that provide this type of care, and these can be found in Appendix B. These longer-duration intensive programs are designed to help clients reestablish recovery routines and prevent further relapses. There should also be an increase in attendance at twelve-step meetings, from a minimum of three meetings per week up to ninety meetings in ninety days.

LEVEL OF CARE FIVE (LOC 5)

LOC 5 is the most intensive and demanding level of care. It includes inpatient treatment at a specialized facility for four to six weeks or longer. This level of care necessitates a disruption of daily life and may have a significant impact on a job or career. However, as disruptive as inpatient treatment is, if a person does not respond to other, less intrusive levels of care, inpatient treatment may be the best option.

Inpatient treatment can be especially helpful for clients who have more than one out-of-control addiction. Common co-occurring forms of addictions include alcohol or other drugs, gambling, and eating disorders. Inpatient and residential treatment centers provide the best opportunity for dealing with multiple addictions together, which is imperative for successful recovery.

The success of inpatient treatment, as with all levels of care, is largely dependent on the willingness of the sex addict to participate actively in his or her treatment and assume responsibility for his or her recovery. Treatment for sex addiction is not a passive process. It requires the addict to work, listen, learn, follow, and ultimately surrender to the treatment process. There are excellent facilities that provide this type of care. A list is found in Appendix B. An integral part of inpatient treatment is attending twelve-step meetings. After treatment, the client should attend at least three meetings a week for six months, and thereafter not less than two meetings per week. Some have a goal of attending ninety meetings in the first ninety days after discharge.

At each level of care, the sex addict must examine his or her total recovery plan and identify gaps and deficiencies. These typically include not making twelve-step meetings a priority, not having or not meeting consistently with a sponsor, or not having contact with the addict's Circle of Five. There may also be an absence of other recovery routines that support recovery. An examination of the recovering addict's life will likely show that he or she had been engaging in questionable behaviors for a time prior to the slip or relapse. To sum up:

LOC 1

• One individual therapy session per week.

• Two twelve-step meetings per week.

LOC 2

• Two individual therapy sessions per week. Some clients may require more therapy, up to one session each day.

• A minimum of three twelve-step meetings a week, with consideration given to a 90/90.

• The increased therapy schedule should continue for three to six weeks or more, depending on how the client responds.

LOC 3

- Brief intensive outpatient treatment, such as the Hope & Freedom Three-Day Intensive program. This level of care should include a polygraph exam.

- A minimum of three twelve-step meetings a week, with consideration given to a 90/90.

LOC 4

- Intensive outpatient treatment for one to three weeks.

- Minimum of three twelve-step meeting per week, with consideration given to a 90/90.

LOC 5

- Inpatient treatment at a specialized facility for four to six weeks.

- Minimum of three twelve-step meetings per week for six months, with consideration given to a 90/90, and then no fewer than two meetings per week.

Consequences of a Slip or Relapse

Orville's Story

Orville's acting-out behavior had been limited to viewing Internet pornography and compulsive masturbation. Rather than minimize his addiction, Orville worked hard in recovery, attending several meetings each week, meeting with his sponsor, and having a weekly therapy session. After three years in recovery from sex addiction, Orville was feeling good about his recovery. Since he was sure he was doing well, he stopped attending twelve-step meetings and quit meeting with his sponsor. Orville was sure that he was cured, and confident that he would not go back to his old behavior.

He withdrew $50,000 from his retirement account for a remodeling project on his house. Soon after making the withdrawal he found the project was going to be delayed for a few weeks. He kept the money *in a separate account so it would not be spent. But when his wife went out of town for a few days, he decided to call an escort service and agreed to pay the person $500 for a "date."*

Over the next several weeks he gradually acquired the habit of paying for sex, until he was acting out every week. He liked the idea of sleeping with what he considered to be high-class women who demanded $1,000 or more. Orville did not keep track of the money he spent because he thought he could replace it before it was missed. However, as a surprise, his wife agreed to move ahead with the remodeling project and needed the money to pay the contractor. She discovered that that the entire $50,000 had been spent. Of even greater concern was the fact she uncovered that he had withdrawn an additional $50,000 and had already spent most of it. She demanded that Orville move out of the house and filed for divorce.

What are the consequences of relapse? One possibility is divorce. If a divorce is the best immediately identifiable option, I recommend postponing it rather than putting an immediate end to the marriage because other steps may be taken to redeem the addict and save the marriage. If the partner chooses not to divorce, additional boundaries must be set and reinforced with the addict. The addict will know the partner can still initiate divorce at any time. The partner should communicate the gravity of the situation to the addict by taking explicit steps to respond to the acting out. In this scenario, the addict is not being punished for being "bad"; he or she is learning (again) that any sexually acting-out behavior has consequences.

I am hesitant for couples to separate right away in response to a relapse, because I believe that once a couple is living apart it is difficult to get them to reconcile. An alternative to separation involving different residences is a separation within the same home. If space is available, the sex addict could move into an empty bedroom with restricted access to the partner's restroom and dressing area. If an extra bedroom is not available, the addict could sleep on a sofa in a different room, or get a cot or sleeping bag and sleep on the other side of the bedroom.

Another consequence of a slip or relapse is the additional expense of more intensive treatment. Treatment is not a punishment; it is a consequence of acting out. Financial setbacks to the family brought on by a slip or a relapse should impact the addict the most. For example, this may mean that following a slip or a relapse, an addict needs to forgo recreational pursuits and restrict personal expenditures. For some men, it may mean getting rid of a hunting lease, selling a boat, or forgoing season tickets to sporting events. For some women it might mean an end to personal shoppers or health club memberships. For addicts of either gender it might entail selling a luxury vehicle and purchasing a used vehicle that is the minimum necessary for his or her transportation needs.

Another significant potential consequence may be for the addict to sign a *post-nuptial* agreement as a condition for the partner staying with the sex addict. This agreement would state that if the marriage ends from any *future* acting out, the addict will walk away from the marriage with fewer of the assets accumulated in the relationship. Executing a legal document with a bad behavior clause is a radical step. But if the marriage is to continue after a relapse, the partner needs to know that the sex addict is serious about staying in recovery.

If the partner accepts the sex addict without any consequences, what will motivate change? The addict might believe he or she can continue acting out and merely appear sorry if caught again. Thus, it is essential for the partner to set boundaries that include clear consequences in the event of a relapse.

CHAPTER 16

A BLUEPRINT FOR REBUILDING BROKEN TRUST

When a couple first determines that they are going to have a relationship together, they give spontaneously, and extend and receive trust. Engaging in an intimate relationship is itself an act of trust. The exchange of trust is not earned; it is a reciprocal commitment that takes place when two people fall in love. Some find that love and trust are so intertwined that they find it difficult to separate the two.

I like to think of this as a "trust bucket." The bucket is relatively full as the relationship develops. Deposits are continually made into the trust bucket that help to strengthen and add value to the relationship.

When trust is breached, relationships are shaken to their core. The trust bucket is quickly drained and ends up empty. If there is no trust, what reason is there to continue loving?

Trust is slowly rebuilt over a period of time. There is an understandable impatience on the part of sex addicts in recovery when their spouse does not show high levels of trust after a few weeks or months of recovery. The man will frequently ask, "Doesn't she realize I am doing good recovery work?" Or in her case, "When is he going to trust me again?"

Trust can be rebuilt when there is reason to trust your partner again. It is understandable not to trust that person until you see evidence of solid recovery in action. Do not be trapped into believing that you must squelch your misgivings and suspicions because your partner says, "You have to believe me. I'm not acting out anymore!" You want to believe the recovering sex addict, but remember the past lies and the broken promises.

Disclosure and a successful polygraph do not necessarily rebuild trust. However, a truthful disclosure may patch the hole in the trust bucket. Honesty during a disclosure can lay the foundation for rebuilding trust. But the bucket is still empty. The couple can begin again making deposits into the trust bucket, and with enough effort on the part of the recovering addict and his/her partner, it is possible for trust to eventually be fully restored.

How Do You Rebuild Trust?

Believe what you see. If your partner is doing the work of recovery and you see continued evidence of this, perhaps there is reason to begin to have trust again. While it is not healthy for you to be in the role of checking up on your partner like a detective, you will soon see evidence that he or she is or is not worthy of trust.

Believe your feelings. Learn once again to listen to your inner voice. Unfortunately, many partners have learned not to trust their feelings because the sex addict was so convincing in the past. He or she may have gone to extraordinary lengths to persuade you not to trust your feelings. In the past you denied suspicions and dismissed the inner voice telling you that something was going on behind your back. You convinced yourself it was all in your mind, or your partner convinced you to trust his or her version of the truth and not your own reality. Part of taking care of yourself is realizing that you can trust your feelings and your inner voice.

You now have reason to be suspicious of behavior that does not fit your partner's normal activities, or when there are gaps in what he or she tells you. When you see changes in his or her work schedule, spending habits, or any area that causes you to wonder what else might be going on, you have a right to answers. If suspicions prove to be unfounded, you can let go of your uneasiness. If later you have questions about his or her behavior, you have a right to ask questions to get the information you need in order to know whether your partner is continuing in recovery or is in the process of returning to active addiction. As you find your partner keeping commitments, continuing meeting with a therapist and sponsor, attending twelve-step meetings, and acting in a trustworthy manner, you can slowly begin trusting your partner again.

Never again will you trust him or her just because you love that person or because your partner is convincing. You find that you can trust your partner's actions based on what you can verify. Trust can return and even become stronger than before when you have a concrete foundation for it, and not just a belief that you should be trusting.

When Ronald Reagan was America's president, his signature phrase for relations with the former Soviet Union was "Trust but verify." What makes sense in negotiations between countries also makes sense as you seek to rebuild trust in your relationship: Trust but verify. Rely on what you can see. Believe what you know to be true. Have confidence in your partner's recovery *when you see* the evidence of recovery. Your trust will no longer be predicated on your partner sounding believable, but on him or her proving daily to be trustworthy.

Following disclosure, set up a process to keep the relationship free of secrets and provide an atmosphere in which trust can be rebuilt. There are two concrete tools that help accomplish this. The first is a weekly check-in that the recovering sex addict does with his or her partner called the FASTT Check-in. The second is to set a schedule of follow-up polygraph exams. The work done in recovery to this point has succeeded in halting the depletion of the trust bucket. Now you are making deposits into your trust bucket, which takes time. Be patient and concentrate on the basics of solid recovery.

FASTT Check-in Process

A FASTT Check-in is a brief weekly process where the addict gives his or her partner a progress report concerning recovery. The purpose of the FASTT Check-in is to keep the partner informed about the addict's recovery activities, normalize talking about recovery-related topics, and allow both partners to be alert for signs that recovery needs to receive greater priority. In FASTT, F is for Feelings, A is for Activities in recovery, S is for a sexual Sobriety statement or Slip report, the first T is for Threats, and the last T is for Tools.

FASTT Check-ins should continue for at least three years following disclosure, or if there has been a slip or relapse, until three years of continuous recovery has been established. Check-ins are ongoing during this period and are the *responsibility of the sex addict to initiate*. Most check-ins can be done in ten minutes or less. If there is a slip involved or there has been evasive behavior, the check-in may require additional time.

The couple needs to set the day and time for the check-in. A good time for the check-in is an evening when both partners can engage in recovery work. For example, an excellent time would be when the husband and the wife both attend a twelve-step meeting or at the end of a day when both have an individual therapy session. Once they have agreed on the schedule, there should be a commitment from both partners to make this a standing appointment. If one is traveling, the appointment should be kept by phone. The FASTT Check-in format should be followed for each check-in.

FEELINGS

The check-in begins with the sex addict talking about his or her feelings at the present time. If multiple feelings are present, the sex addict should try to get in touch with each, stating them to the partner. Feelings checks are especially important for men, because often men relegate their feelings to a small handful such as mad, happy, or sad.

Some men have grown up with the understanding that "real men" do not show a wide range of feelings. They may have been put down by a parent or a peer for displays of emotions not considered "manly." As a result, they may need to practice learning to express their feelings and to let their partner know what they are experiencing. This is particularly true when experiencing fear, hurt, or shame. Because these are feelings that express vulnerability, they are difficult for many men to allow themselves to feel and to share. The weekly feelings check-in procedure helps a man get in touch with his emotional life.

ACTIVITIES IN RECOVERY[35]

In this part of the check-in, the recovering sex addict has the opportunity to talk about all of the things he or she completed that week to support recovery. If the individual is actively working on recovery, the list will be extensive. Some activities that will be included are therapy sessions, both individual and group, and attendance at twelve-step meetings. While the recovering sex addict cannot talk about the work that others do in twelve-step meetings, he can tell his partner about the work he does at meetings. While a detailed list of recovery activities provides the partner a degree of comfort, the sex addict should recognize that this list is not meant to impress the partner but rather to communicate the week's activities in recovery. Recovery is both a state of mind and a set of actions. Though the addict may say he or she is in a recovery state of mind, the partner has no way to validate it. However, a recitation of the sex addict's actual recovery activities lends credence to the assertion that the addict is working toward change and recovery.

Another category of recovery-related activities involves accountability to others. Early in recovery, the recovering sex addict should be meeting weekly with a sponsor. During meetings the sponsor gets a report of how the sex addict has progressed during the week as well as a chance to review given assignments. The sponsor's job is to mentor the sex addict and guide him or her through the Twelve Steps of recovery. This will take at least several months, and it is common for it to take a year or two and sometimes longer. During this time there are frequent reading and writing assignments. The sex addict should be able to give a report to his or her partner of the work done with his or her sponsor. Twelve-step work is highly personal, and the recovering sex addict needs to do assignments in private, but not in secret. He or she needs to work on any written assignments the sponsor gives without having to reveal the specific contents of what he or she writes.

This may seem like it counters the desire to put secrets to an end, but it does not. Secrets must end, but each person has a right to privacy. For example, when a person closes the door upon entering a bathroom, he or she is asking not for secrecy but for privacy. Recovery work requires a sex addict to delve into the long-hidden dark recesses of memory and experience.

In the same way, the sex addict should be allowed to participate in therapy and to do work in session with the therapist with privacy about what takes place in the session. The exercises he or she is involved in, the details of what is discussed, and any journal entries made should be kept private as the recovering sex addict completes the process. Privacy around twelve-step work and therapy are crucial for recovery.

As described early in this book, not only is the sex addict accountable to a particular sponsor, but he or she should also have other persons to whom he or she is accountable.

During the check-in with the partner, the sex addict should be able to talk about various contacts with persons who hold him or her accountable, such as a sponsor and the Circle of Five. The contacts with these entrusted people will keep recovery a priority.

Another recovery activity is reading recovery-related books and literature. Most twelve-step fellowships provide publications that explain their recovery program as well as offering stories about people who have followed their program to achieve successful recovery. There are many books about sex addiction recovery that may be part of an addict's weekly reading. Sustained recovery includes reading recovery-related material weekly. A helpful practice is to keep a recovery book on the nightstand and to read it on a daily basis.

SEXUAL SOBRIETY STATEMENT OR SLIP REPORT

The next part of the check-in is a sexual sobriety statement or a slip report. The sexual sobriety statement includes the sexual sobriety date (the day after the last episode of sexual acting out), as well as the fact that the addict has been sexually sober since the last check-in. For example, the individual might say, "I have been sexually sober from all acting-out behaviors for the past week. And I have had continuous sexual sobriety since February 7 of last year." A slip *of any kind* is reported. And by definition, if there has been a slip, then there is no sexual sobriety. They are mutually exclusive.

THREATS

In earlier chapters, the word *trigger* was used because it accurately describes what the sex addict faces. Sex Addicts Anonymous's "Green Book" defines triggers as "any situation or behavior that causes us to feel a powerful desire to act out."[36] However, using the word *trigger* in the check-in often communicates to the partner that acting out is imminent. Experiencing triggers is a normal part of recovery. Their presence does not mean that an addict is teetering on the brink of losing sexual sobriety.

To better communicate what the addict faces daily, I use the word *threat* to describe situations that place the recovering addict at potential risk and require the application of recovery tools. Threats are a part of daily life for everyone. For example, staying in the sun too long presents the threat of developing skin cancer. Every time we get into an automobile, we should scan for conditions that could be a threat to safety and watch for threats from other drivers.

Sex addicts should get in the habit of continually doing a threat assessment to guard against things that endanger their recovery. Threats are normal in recovery. There may be visual threats as well as emotional ones. There are also threats because of job stress or some crisis in life. During check-in, the addict should feel free to talk about threats he or she encounters. In fact, if threats are seldom shared during a check-in, it would be safe to assume that the reason for the silence is not that there were no threats, but that the addict did not feel the threats could be shared. The more the check-in process becomes routine, the freer sex addicts will be to share the threats they experience.

Sex addicts are advised to share the threats in a way that is not traumatizing to their partner. For example, each day there are visual threats to a sex addict. In his check-in he does not say, "I had a visual threat at work today. There is a new employee who has long, dark hair . . ." This is needlessly traumatizing to the partner. Rather, he should say, "For visual threats this week I used the following tools . . ." Nothing more about the specifics of visual threats is added. When a person is in solid recovery, visual threats are a matter of course each day. But they are dealt with effectively by utilizing tools to maintain sexual sobriety.

Another common threat that happens every week for sex addicts is that of intrusive thoughts. Intrusive thoughts may be the beginning of a sexual fantasy, the memory of a previous acting-out experience, a sexual dream, or the memory of a pornographic image or video. It would be traumatizing to the partner to talk specifically about each intrusive thought. (I tell partners that if they could get inside the mind of a sex addict for even a few seconds, they would immediately want out.) Rather, they say, "For intrusive thoughts this week I used the following tools . . ."

TOOLS[37]

If threats were shared and the check-in ended at that point, the partner would be naturally and unavoidably concerned. After each type of threat is shared, the addict should discuss what tools were used to respond. A good practice is to share one threat at a time and to verbally list what tool was used to address that threat.

Throughout recovery, sex addicts learn a variety of effective methods for responding to threats. Some of these tools are learned in therapy and twelve-step groups. The tools may be as simple as breaking visual contact, followed by engaging in another activity to take the addict's mind off the threat. Other tools may involve changing one's schedule to allow for attendance at additional twelve-step meetings. The addict may call a sponsor or someone in recovery for immediate support, or schedule an extra therapy session to process a threatening event and to prepare for handing similar future situations.

ADDITIONAL ITEMS

The check-in may include other items mutually agreed upon, such as accountability for time and money or a safety plan for travel. Any additional items that the couple wishes to include are at their discretion. At a minimum, the five points of the FASTT Check-in described here should be followed. Some wounded partners later choose to also do a check-in with their sex-addicted partner. They check in about the recovery work they are doing with regard to healing and to dealing with their trauma, along with any unwanted behaviors they are working to eliminate. For the first year of check-ins, I recommend that the check-in be only one-way, with the sex addict checking in with the partner.

The Partner's Response

The partner's response to the check-in is crucial in order for the process to be successful. Her or his role is to provide a safe place for the recovering sex addict to talk about recovery. To accomplish this, the partner needs to do three things that may not initially feel natural or comfortable.

1. Listen to the check-in completely, without interruption.

2. Do not ask questions.

3. When the addict is through with the check-in, thank him or her, and hug. But what if the partner is not comfortable or ready to hug the addict? That certainly happens, and partners may withhold hugs initially if they feel they are not ready for this. My intent is to move a couple toward breaking through the touch barrier. After a serious breach of trust, some partners find that first step of touching their partner extremely difficult. It is recommended that partners break through the touch barrier when they are able.

Yet, perhaps the most difficult part of this process is not asking questions. It is natural for a partner who hears there were visual threats to say, "What did you actually see? I don't understand." In truth, men and women are threatened in different ways. A significant source of threats to recovery for men is visual stimuli. A wife does not need to understand why her husband was threatened. She needs to accept the fact that he was threatened and felt he needed to share that experience during the check-in.

It is natural for a partner to want to know specifics about threats. And some want the details about where the visual threats took place, who the person was, and what she or he looked like, as well as additional details. It may be normal to want this level of detail, but it is very injurious to the partner. What you can know is that there are threats in abundance every day. If your sex-addicted partner is using tools to counter the threats, you can be assured that those potential threats do not endanger your relationship. The addict's recognition of threats and use of tools is a good indicator that he or she is in solid recovery.

The next morning, if the partner wants additional details about something shared at the check-in, she or he may ask for details. The tone of questioning, as well as the attitude during this process, impacts how safe the addict feels about the check-in the following week. But again, the questions should not be about specifics around visual threats or intrusive thoughts.

FASTT CHECK-IN

Weekly Check-in with Partner

1. Determine day and time for the check-in. Make this a standing appointment and keep it!

2. Check-in is the responsibility of the sex addict to initiate.

3. The purpose of the FASTT Check-in is to keep the partner informed as to recovery activities, normalize talking about recovery-related topics, and allow both partners to be alert for signs that recovery needs to receive greater priority.

4. Follow **FASTT** format:

   • **F**eelings check.

   > What are you feeling at present? If multiple feelings are present, try to get in touch with each one, naming them out loud to your partner.

   • **A**ctivities in recovery.

   > The heart of this part of the check-in is to share about recovery activities utilizing the Recovery Points System—a method of tracking a person's recovery by assigning recovery points to common recovery activities. The addict repeats three sentences that are related to the Recovery Points System.[38]

   > I am in the _____ recovery phase.

   > My weekly recovery points goal is _____.

   > This week I earned _____ recovery points doing the following activities. (The addict then reads from his or her completed Recovery Points Worksheet.)

   • **S**obriety statement or **S**lip report (if instances of predisclosure acting out are remembered, those details are shared at this time).

> A statement about your sexual sobriety, such as "I have not acted out since my last check-in and have been sexually sober since _____."

> If there has been a slip, it should be revealed in detail at this time.

- **Threats.** (Both "T"s are worked at the same time.)

- **Tools** you used to respond to each threat. (Tools are anything that is used to counter a threat. Examples of tools would include calling your sponsor, journaling, praying, reciting a poem or a favorite quote or Scripture, singing—anything that is used to move the addict away from the threat at hand.)

> What threats have you identified since the last check-in?

> Example: "For visual threats this week I used the following tool(s) . . ."

> Example: "For intrusive thoughts this week I used the following tool(s) . . ."

   Important: Do not give more details than this about these two types of threats; to do so needlessly traumatizes your partner.

> Example: "I was stressed at work this week and used [name of recovery tool] to deal with it."

5. The check-in can also include other items as mutually agreed upon, such as accountability for time and money or safety plan for travel.

PARTNER'S RESPONSIBILITY— CREATE A COCOON/ZONE OF SAFETY

1. Listen all the way through the check-in without interruption.

2. Don't ask questions.

3. When your partner is through, thank him or her and hug him or her. (If partner still has questions the next day, he or she can ask.)

Follow-up Polygraph Exams

An important tool for keeping secrets at bay is for the sex addict to have follow-up polygraph exams periodically. These are similar to the baseline polygraph, but the questions are designed to learn how well the sex addict is doing in recovery. There is no attempt to gather further information predating the baseline polygraph.

Recovery is a lifelong process that requires ongoing attention in order for it to be maintained successfully. After the initial recovery work with a rigorous aftercare program, I encourage clients to have additional Aftercare Intensives every six months and up to three years after they enter recovery, and annually after that. Each Aftercare Intensive includes the opportunity for a follow-up polygraph exam.

Addiction, according to the "Big Book" of Alcoholics Anonymous,[39] is "cunning, baffling, and powerful." Sex addiction is no exception. Even when recovery is going well, there may be subtle temptations to act out. The knowledge that a polygraph is scheduled helps to focus the mind and restore sanity long enough for a sex addict to be able to break free from the pull of the addiction and make choices consistent with recovery. Follow-up polygraph exams are great tools because the sex addict can use them for additional motivation in his or her recovery. They are also most useful to help the individual become a person of honesty and integrity in every area of personal and professional life.

A wonderful benefit of follow-up polygraph exams is restored trust in the relationship. Rather than having to rely solely on a recovering addict's self-report that he or she is not acting out, the partner has proof that the addict is telling the truth. It is not enough to know that the addict is in recovery and all previous acting-out behavior has been revealed. Follow-up polygraph exams provide objective, accurate, up-to-date information that confirms that the sexual acting out has ended—or not. There may be initial resistance on the part of couples to use ongoing polygraph exams. Some protest that they should have trust without them. However, once trust is breached, what is the basis for restoring it? Experience with sex addicts shows that trust without proof is not advisable in that it can be a setup for further betrayal.

Some say that polygraph exams used this way are a crutch, and an effort should be made as soon as possible to get rid of the crutch. However, sometimes people need to use crutches to walk. Is that not preferable to falling? Moreover, rather than seeing polygraph exams as crutches, I view them as tools. They are effective in rebuilding trust in a relationship. They have inestimable value in helping to further motivate sex addicts to learn new recovery-oriented thoughts and behaviors.

Scheduling follow-up polygraph exams is the responsibility of the addict. The partner should not have to remind the addict that a polygraph exam is due, just as it is not the job of the therapist to make sure that the recovering addict knows when an exam needs to be scheduled.

Follow-up polygraph exams are good occasions for celebration. The celebration is not for the fact that the exam has been passed, but for achieving another recovery milestone. It is a time of celebration that the relationship has been restored as much as it has been to this point, and that it is on the road to potential full restoration.

As in the case of the baseline polygraph exam, there are four relevant questions on the exam. These questions are crafted by the therapist and the partner. The following are examples of questions that may be asked on the follow-up polygraph exam. All of these questions are time-limited in that they ask about behavior that has occurred since the previous exam.

Since your last polygraph exam:

• Have you been sexual with anyone other than your spouse?

• Have you had any contact with any former sex partner? (If there is occasion to see former partners during the normal course of life, the question could be "Other than what you have revealed, have you had any contact with any former sex partner?")

- Have you engaged in any "grooming" behavior? (Grooming is not necessarily the same thing as flirting, though flirting is a grooming behavior. Grooming is doing or saying anything that is intended to see if the possibility for a future relationship exists.)

- Have you engaged in any cybersex behaviors?

- Have you intentionally viewed any pornography? (The definition of pornography here includes anything that is sought out to stimulate or bring about sexual arousal.)

- Have you patronized any sex-oriented businesses?

- Have you acted out sexually in any way?

There may be other questions that the partner wants included. Sometimes there may be a particular incident that is troubling, about which she or he feels the need for additional information. As a rule the questions are broad enough to cover any sexual behavior that does not include the partner. However, if the partner needs to ask a specific question, she or he is able to do so.

Success in recovery depends on sex addicts taking responsibility for all of their behavior. If they succeed in recovery, it is because they have done the work and taken the actions necessary to bring it about. If they fail, they cannot blame their partners, therapists, or sponsors. It cannot be stated more clearly: The sex addict is the only one who can succeed at the work of recovery and achieve freedom from his or her sex addiction.

Healing Specific to Marriages Where the Husband Is a Sex Addict

One thing recovering male sex addicts who are married have in common is that they want their wife to heal from her trauma. They may not think of it in those terms. To be sure, men suffering from sex addiction are still so self-centered early in recovery that the only thing that matters to them is how *they* feel. They desperately want their wives to "get over it." They want their wives to stop bringing up the past and recognize the progress they are making in recovery.

Sex addicts do not always realize this is self-centered. What they do know is that as they may be working hard to stay in recovery and live a life of integrity, their wives may not seem to be making as much progress. There are times when it seems like the wife takes a couple of steps forward and then bumps into trauma triggers and takes a large step backward. She is still moving forward, but the presence of trauma triggers understandably slows her progress. Do you have the patience necessary to see your wife through until she is completely healed from the wounds that you have caused? How long do you need to be patient? Just as long as it takes. Her healing will not happen quickly, and her healing will not follow a predictable path. Some women heal quicker than others.

The alternative is that you lose patience with her or get angry at her for bringing up the past. You determine that she is just trying to make you feel bad and that she does not want to get better. So under the influence of your lack of patience, you angrily say, "Fine. You can keep living in the past if you want to. I'm getting better and you just can't see it." And you disconnect from her emotionally and concentrate solely on your recovery.

What is the result? You may continue to do pretty well in your recovery. But your wife will still be wounded—and she may remain that way for many years. She will still be suffering the effects of the trauma that you caused and that you now expect her to just "get over." You will continue to wish your relationship was better, but you will not be able to see how to get the two of you to a better place.

The problem is not that you are not doing solid recovery work. The problem is that your wife is still very wounded. Are you able to put your self-centeredness aside long enough for her to heal? Can you quit being the self-centered demigod you have been and realize that your acting-out behavior has shattered her as though she were a china plate?

Yet you have treated her as though she were made of some resilient, unbreakable material.

How long will it take for a woman to heal from the trauma caused by her sex addict partner? The answer depends on how involved in the healing process the husband is. If he is not involved and expects his wife to just "get over it," full healing may not come for many years. Sometimes women continue to feel the impact of their trauma decades later.

But in those cases where the husband is as committed to his wife's healing as he is to his own recovery, a significant amount of healing can take place in the first year. Full healing will take longer, perhaps three to five years, and in some cases longer. But the fact remains that a lot of healing can take place during the first twelve months of recovery.

Both of you must be willing to pursue your own recovery. That includes each of you attending twelve-step meetings, working with sponsors, and, if you can afford it, each of you working with a therapist. Your own recovery must have a solid foundation before you can hope to do very much in the way of couples work. After each of you has done significant work in individual recovery, you will be ready to work with a couples therapist. Many couples want to plunge immediately into couples therapy. But traditional couples therapy needs to wait until both of you have a solid base in your individual recoveries. (Note: Intensive outpatient programs, like the Three-Day Intensives offered at Hope & Freedom and other providers, are able to speed this process along.)

At the same time, you must be willing to lower your expectations and allow your wife to heal at her own pace. There are additional things you can do that will help with this process:

• Be patient.
• Take ownership of your behavior. ("I was wrong." "I hurt you." "You didn't deserve what I did.")

- In the same way, there are things you can do that will hinder your wife's healing. These include, but are not limited to:

- Getting angry.

- Withdrawing.

- Continuing to be self-centered (making everything all about you).

- Attempting to do damage control by minimizing or denying past acting-out behavior.

What Else Does She Need?

Let's say that you really work at helping your wife heal. You start putting her interests ahead of your own. You become less self-centered. Phrases like "I was wrong" and "You didn't deserve that" are less alien to you. What else does she need from you for the relationship to be restored?

One of the things I hear from women in most of the Intensives that I conduct is that they want to know that they really matter to their partner. They have heard the things he has done as part of his acting out. Sometimes they hear about the extraordinary lengths their partner went to in order to impress an acting-out partner. They want to know why they cannot have the same romance in their marriage. They want to feel that they are special enough to their husband that he would want to go out of his way to make them feel special. I've heard two women use the same old-fashioned phrase recently, about ten days apart. Both of them said, "I want him to court me." Courtship did not go out of style with windmills and buggy whips.

One word of caution. While your wife may truly want you to court her, she may not be in a position right now to accept romantic overtures from you. That does not mean she will never be at that place. It just means you continue to look for opportunities to show her that you love her, even if she is not in an emotional position to show you that she appreciates your attention.

How do you court your wife? There are lots of ways to show that you care. Flowers, gifts, love notes, and the like may not be things she is ready for now, but the time will come when she will appreciate them. This time when you initiate these expressions of love, do not stop them the way you did when you got engaged or got married. You need to be willing to continue these expressions of love and affection throughout your lifetime together.

When is the last time you planned a date with your wife? For many guys the idea of a date is dinner and/or a movie, with the wife making all of the arrangements and picking the restaurant. All the guy does is show up and think she should be happy to have him around.

Suppose you were single now and met your wife for the first time. In order to win her to be your one true love, you would be pretty creative in the dating department. Capture that same creativity now and get outside your comfort zone and plan things that she would enjoy.

One man told me how much his wife enjoyed going to hot rod rallies and tractor pulls. I thought I would test that in a couples session I had later. When I asked his wife if she enjoyed these things, she said that what she enjoyed was being with her husband. And if it meant doing the things that he enjoyed, she was willing to do them so they could have some time together.

I asked her what were the things that she enjoyed most. After a bit of thought, she said she enjoyed concerts and taking long walks in the woods. When I asked her to recall the last time she had done either with her husband, she could not remember. Her husband was shocked. He said he did not know that she liked going to concerts. And he could not remember her ever telling him that she liked to take walks in the woods. Then his wife remarked, "You never asked."

What are the things that your wife enjoys doing? Are there special places where she likes to go but you have not been to in a while? If she could go anyplace that she wanted, where would that place be? What was the date she had with you at any time in the past that she enjoyed the most?

This would be a good time to make a list of things that your wife enjoys doing. What are her favorite activities? What do you think she would enjoy doing if she were not always trying to fit into your schedule? Would she enjoy taking a cooking lesson with you? How about attending a dog show together? Would she enjoy taking a day trip to a nearby city?

One of the ways to show that you care for her is to make sure to remember special calendar dates. Birthdays, anniversaries, and Valentine's Day are among the days you know are important to her. But there are other dates that are also important. Has she ever reminded you of the anniversary of your first date? Or does she seem to recall the day you proposed as much as she does the day you got married?

Some other dates that are not highlights for her but are still on her mind are either dates that correspond with some past acting-out behavior or dates when she discovered your behavior. While these are not dates that either of you want to celebrate, you can know that they are dates she may not be able to forget. As a guy, you may think (or hope) that as long as she does not bring these dates up, then she has forgotten them. However, this is unlikely; more often than not, these dates are significant trauma triggers.

One woman told me that she vividly remembers the day her husband called to tell her he would never come home again. She related the agony that she went through as she tried to make sense of why he was leaving her. Every year she said she remembers that date and wishes her husband would at least acknowledge the fact that she still hurts as she remembers that phone call and the events that followed.

Recently a woman told me that she wished her husband would remember her in some way on Mother's Day. He was shocked when she said that. He said, "But you are not a mother!" That was true, but his wife went on to tell him how it was a day that she dreaded because many other women were celebrating and she just had to pretend that day was not really important. She told him, "I just wish you could give me a card on that day that told me how much you love me!"

Do Not Settle

Do not settle for less than a happy marriage. It may not seem possible right now for your marriage to be restored. Some people may think it would take a miracle for their marriage ever to be healed. But miracles do happen. In the final analysis, for your relationship to be restored it will take both of you working individually and together. Both of you need to be willing to do the very difficult work of recovery. And both of you need to be willing to devote as much time and energy as necessary in order to see the relationship restored.

Restoring your relationship will be the most difficult part of the recovery journey. There may be times when you feel it would just be easier to end the relationship and start over. Certainly ending the relationship would be easier in the short term. But if your relationship could be restored and be all that you have hoped it could be, you would probably say it was worth it.

Your relationship can be restored. I have seen it happen with many, many couples. Continuing to do the hard work of recovery can result in the relationship that you want. You will be glad that you made the effort.

CHAPTER 17

SURVEY RESULTS: FACTORS THAT HELPED RESTORE TRUST

At first glance it might appear that this chapter relates more to partners than it does to sex addicts. However, both can benefit from the wisdom shared in these survey results.

If you are a sex addict, I would suggest that you compile a master list of the factors that help and hinder the restoration of trust. I would also reinforce that you keep in mind that restoration of trust will not happen automatically with the passing of time. There are numerous actions you can take that will enhance trust. And there are many other things you can do that will hurt the trust-rebuilding process.

One truth about the rebuilding of trust needs to be recognized. You can do ten things that enhance the trust-rebuilding process. Then you can do one thing that hurts trust and may completely erode any gains that have been made. That may not seem fair, but it is true. You may do many, many things that build trust. But because the trust that your partner had in your relationship has been so fundamentally betrayed, one untrustworthy act can place you back in a trust deficit.

Another truth about trust rebuilding is that the more times trust is eroded, the more difficult it is to reestablish it. If you are new to recovery, this is the time to take stock of how you live and how you interact with your partner. The time to work on trust restoration is today.

Referring back to the survey that 103 partners of sex addicts responded to, participants were asked how they would characterize the level of trust that existed between them and their sex-addicted partner (see Figure 6). Two participants (1.9 percent) said that, at present, they fully trust their partner; twenty-four (23.9 percent) said they have significant trust in their sex-addicted partner; forty (38.8 percent) said they have some trust in their partner; and thirty-seven (35.9 percent) said they have no trust in their partner.

FIGURE 6

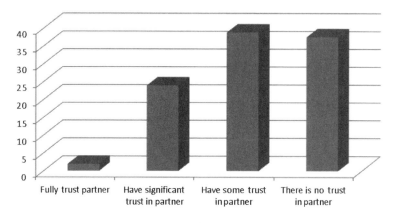

Level of Trust in Relationship?

The first thing that is apparent from this input is that very few respondents fully trust their partners. Indeed, rebuilding trust in a committed relationship after discovery of sexual acting out is extremely difficult. And yet about 64 percent of those who responded to the survey have at least some trust in their partners.

You will notice that many of the factors that respondents indicated helped to restore trust were also listed in Chapter 14 as factors that helped to promote healing. It makes sense that many of the same factors that promote healing also help in the rebuilding of trust—so there is some necessary repetition. It was tempting to eliminate all of these duplications for the sake of brevity. However, repetition is often helpful in the process of learning generally, and I believe this repetition is worthwhile because it emphasizes that in your journey of recovery, many of the same actions you take can promote healing *and* contribute significantly to restoring trust in your relationship. If that is your priority, you will want to learn about what has helped, as well as what has not helped, in rebuilding trust from the experience and wisdom of partners who have walked this path.

You will once again notice that factors some partners found unhelpful in rebuilding trust, such as therapy and attending twelve-step meetings, other partners found to be helpful. You must determine what is most helpful for you. Just because someone else's experience was not helpful to them, that is no reason to dismiss it without giving it a chance to see if it will be helpful in your relationship. Your experience is your own, and may be very different.

When considering the mixed experiences partners reported with regard to twelve-step meetings, you need to determine for yourself the extent to which that resource will be helpful to you. Go to the same meeting at least five times in a row before you discount it and determine that it is not helpful. And if that meeting is not helpful after you have attended it five times, try a different meeting. Each meeting has a somewhat different atmosphere and tone. The great strength of twelve-step meetings lies in helping you realize that you are not alone. Through them you can build a support network that will prove invaluable in your journey.

Partners Who Reported No Trust in the Relationship

Partners in this group have provided helpful insights into why no trust exists in their relationship. Many of the responses are not surprising. However, it is noteworthy that even in this group there were some factors that portend the possibility of trust.

WHAT WAS LEAST BENEFICIAL TO RESTORING TRUST?

- Nine of the respondents in this category reported that what most adversely affected trust was their partner's continuing to act out. For some, there was the recognition that the sex addict was trying to do recovery and had had a slip or relapse. For the rest, the sex addict just continued acting out, with little change taking place after the initial discovery of the acting out.

- Thirteen of those surveyed in this category said their partner's habitual lying was a hindrance to trust being rebuilt. Some talked about the lying to cover up acting out. Others reported that their partners seemed to lie about most anything. Some of the time they would lie about things that did not really matter. Others spoke about their partner's lies of omission.

That continuing to act out sexually and lie would be harmful to any restoration of trust in the relationship is self-evident. Other responses included these:

- His waiting for and controlling the disclosure process.

- Inconsistent recovery behaviors.

- Reactive behaviors.

- Too early to tell.

- Many professional people have tried to help us, but unless the addict is willing to change, there is little hope for the relationship to be restored.

- Addict "not remembering" to get rid of all email addresses and contact information of former acting-out partners.

- Words of promise to change. I must see the actions.

- When the addict makes excuses not to seek therapy.

- The notion of entirely "separate" individual recovery. My partner blocks me out of his recovery.

- No accountability at times.

- A couple of false starts through the years where he was only half in recovery and full of arrogance and a bad attitude. This heaped damage on the damage already there.

- His inability to devote time to healing our relationship.

- Continuing to be untruthful about finances.

- Treating the viewing of porn like it was nothing. Telling me every man does it.

- Not having a last will and testament the entire time we were together and then creating one that excluded me.

- My husband keeps to himself in the beginning stages of his recovery. I'm left to wonder if it's working. I'm left to wonder all sorts of things.

- I do not feel he realizes how much he has hurt me, and that he has to be a part of the rebuilding process. Just because he feels his acting out has stopped does not mean the repair happens by itself.

- He does not really apologize for the hurt he has caused. He has not gone out of his way to show that he means it. His apology comes across as him having a minor flaw.

- His work schedule often interferes with his attending meetings and counseling sessions. Things go downhill from there, of course.

- Him complimenting me.

- Trust is supposed to come as a result of consistency of positive behavior over time, and sadly, the thing that has been most consistent is my husband's ability to lie to me and unload on me.

- I love him, but I really can't trust him. Not unless something changes.

- Therapy.

- Twelve-step meetings for partners.

- Lack of recovery resources.

- My husband would do polygraph exams but would not do any recovery work. I know it was puzzling that my husband would still come and do the polygraph, but in the end just doing the polygraph accomplished little change in the bigger picture of our marriage and in his recovery.

- With one exception, my spouse has had to "come clean" about something in order to pass his follow-up polygraph exams. His recovery has stalled as he has become complacent about it.

- The return of some actions that serve as warning signs (new email accounts that were never mentioned; the purchase of a new phone that was never discussed; the purchase of an iPad-like device that was never discussed).

- Lack of commitment to recovery and appreciation for the damage his behavior has wrought on our relationship.

- Not having the polygraph exam done along with therapy.

- He never seemed to have full buy-in to the twelve-step process for sex addiction like he had for drugs and alcohol. He seemed to go through the motions of attending meetings. Never sought out literature to help him understand sex addiction.

- Not proactive in recovery; seemed to be only doing what he thought was expected of him.

- Denial that actions were detrimental to his recovery and possible stepping-stones to full acting out, such as masturbation, soft porn, and helping women in his AA group with their recovery. His inability to see for himself the danger of situations that have the potential to sabotage his recovery. When confronted with those things, only when his AA sponsor would agree that it would sabotage his recovery did he give my concerns any weight of being valid.

- The simple fact that he had been at this his entire life and is over sixty years old. I had heard about the "new" person he had become too many times to believe it.

- Relying too much on my husband. He shifts the blame and ignores that we have a problem.

- I wish I had a printout for my husband to hear again what my therapist told him: "Let your wife have the freedom to feel, whether it is positive or sad. Your acting out got you both here, and now you need to be there for her. She has put up with and lived in the carnage of your acting out; the very least you can do for your wife is to own your acting-out behavior and support her through this storm you put her in."

- His depression.

- We were unable to reestablish trust in the relationship because my husband walked out of therapy.

- Following our work together in an intensive outpatient program, he followed the recovery steps set up for us and I was very hopeful that we would survive as a couple. When I had a significant health issue and was in the hospital for an extended period of time, he resumed acting out and virtually destroyed what progress we had made.

- When he gets angry and impatient with me. It is living through all the pain again and opening those wounds.

WHAT WAS MOST BENEFICIAL TO RESTORING TRUST?

For those who reported that there was currently no trust in their relationship, there are still some positive signs that may yet lead to trust being restored.

- Honest, proactive communication from the addict.

- Consistent recovery behaviors.

- Witnessing the addict taking responsibility for his own recovery.

- Seeing the addict leading in exercises and activities given by our therapist.

- Experiencing the addict having a spirit of humility in words and actions toward me and our children.

- Several mentioned the addict being accountable. Here are some of their specific responses.

  - Having him be accountable for where he has been, who he has talked to, and what his schedule is for the week.

  - There was accountability to begin with; however, he had a big relapse and kept it quiet. Now accountability is not much help in restoring trust.

- When he tells the truth and is accountable for his time, money, and whereabouts.

- The polygraph exam helps restore trust.

- Seeing my husband completely submit to God and make his recovery the priority in his life.

- Participating in psychotherapy with him.

- Listening to my husband share his heart and deepest feelings, thoughts, and emotions in life. This did not happen before.

- Seeing and hearing how humble he has become.

- Seeing the pain in his eyes when he tells me how sorry he is.

- Praying together.

- Ongoing polygraph exams will be a fact of life. His unconditional willingness to give me this has been helpful.

- When he comes forward and talks to me. Just letting me know where he is in his journey of recovery. I do not need every detail. I'm a very understanding person when I have some information. I believe information is key.

- Although trust in our relationship is not yet restored, when he attends group meetings or a meeting with our pastor he usually comes home like he has been to a mental chiropractor. His thinking is realigned. His mood is realigned.

- When he goes to his twelve-step meetings, he comes home in a frame of mind to at least show respect for my limits and values.

- I thought that the polygraph was going to be the ultimate answer for building trust, but it ended up being a double-edged sword in my situation. My husband did not talk to me about anything until he went in for each polygraph. That day he would divulge in the presence of our therapist what he had or had not done. He made sure he did not do certain acting-out behaviors, but he did many other things that showed he was not really getting free, and the trust between us was no better.

- Seeing my spouse accept and acknowledge his disease.

- Seeing my spouse begin to work his recovery program of his own volition.

- Having my spouse answer my questions quickly and what appears to be more openly than in the past.

- My partner taking responsibility for his actions.

- Spouse showing remorse.

- Partner wanting to spend time together and taking the initiative to make that happen.

- Him disclosing when he has a "slip," regardless of how minor it is.

- Spouse wanting to share something he has learned about himself in counseling or at a twelve-step meeting.

- Him agreeing to being tested for STDs; all tests were negative.

- Open communication about his addiction and the emotional aspect of the addiction and the recovery process.

- My spouse calling to check in with me often and calling to tell me when he leaves one place to go to another.

- He has attended workshops about the impact of his behavior on me, and he changed his behavior after that.

- It is going to take time more than anything for me to actually begin to trust.

- His disclosure followed by a polygraph helped restore trust.

- He does a weekly check-in that our therapist prescribed.

- I feel more comfortable saying it was a new beginning to start building the trust back. I also felt more trusting when he seemed to care about my feelings after my anger/hurt letter, and he listened to it without interrupting and getting angry and defensive. The intimacy exercises and the FASTT Check-in when we are doing them help build trust. But unfortunately, it comes crashing down when he stops these.

- My husband being open and honest with me about his past and current thoughts, feelings, and actions.

- He always tries to put my mind at ease.

It is encouraging that even in this group of partners who say there is no trust, many have indicated a process taking place that gives the promise of hope being restored some day.

Partners Who Reported Some Trust in the Relationship
A shortcoming of the survey is that there is no metric that was used by the partners to quantify "some trust." This notwithstanding, it is significant that so many respondents indicated that some trust has been restored in the relationship.

WHAT WAS LEAST BENEFICIAL TO RESTORING TRUST?
- Finding out on my own about his acting out.

- Being told by a trained sex addiction therapist that I had to do whatever it took to work through my major trust issues so that I wouldn't keep voicing my "irrational" thoughts that my spouse was still lying, which turned out to be the case.

- My husband's therapist telling him that I'm co-addicted, that I'm half the problem, that I have somehow caused or enabled his addiction.

- Him getting impatient and avoiding answering my questions.

- Knowing the past and how little I really knew then, and realizing that it could happen again and again.

- Full disclosure, meaning knowing exactly what or who my partner has been looking at.

- Recognizing that the addiction cannot be cured and that it will always be a part of him, and therefore a part of our relationship.

- Husband's inconsistency with recovery activities.

- Husband's inability to answer questions about some activities in the past because he supposedly just doesn't remember.

- Petty lies and general lack of real communication.

- Fruitless apologies with intense remorse but disconnected from change.

- Several mentioned that their partners having to travel for their work is a major problem in rebuilding trust. Here are some of their specific comments:

  - My husband travels, and this is where he has been sexually active outside our marriage. He refuses to be accountable to me when he reaches his hotel, when he gets back in, who he has been out with. He lives life as if he is not accountable to me as his wife. He believes I should trust him just because he says I should when he has lied, deceived, connived, and conned me for over thirty years.

  - My husband travels but has refused to put together a travel plan as his therapist directed.

- He does not put recovery first in his life.

- He is angry and resentful toward me.

- The addict lecturing me and trying to control my recovery.
- Finding out at a polygraph exam that he has not told me the whole truth.
- Finding large purchases made with cash that I didn't know about until afterward.
- His defensiveness when I ask questions and turning it around to make the argument my fault.
- He has no patience with me.
- Reading books on being a better wife. It was too easy to start blaming myself, especially when the books do not take addiction into consideration.
- Not communicating with me.
- Knowing he has dropped out of important groups and church.
- My husband not being consistent about ongoing recovery work.
- The "dribbling out" of information regarding his sexual behaviors/ acting out.
- Ongoing acting-out cycles by my spouse after treatment opportunities.
- My spouse maintaining a victim role and being angry about the time required for healing.
- My spouse felt that we should be "out of this" about six weeks after our intensive outpatient work. He is frustrated that I am not over it yet.
- In the beginning (the first year of recovery), my spouse wasn't consistent with meetings and had a relapse. That set us back.
- Him telling me he is going to change. I needed proof, which only time and polygraph exams have been able to provide.
- My husband sees a therapist who is not trained to work with sex addicts, and I feel she is not the best choice. I feel she does not push him enough.

- Not working his steps with a sponsor.

- Me giving in to negative feelings and thoughts.

- When my husband acts out or has a slip.

- When he participates in behaviors that could lead to acting out, such as flirting with women, looking at women like they are objects, drinking, and staying out late with friends or coworkers.

- When he lies to me about big and small things. When he says he will do something (pack the kids' lunches, for example) and doesn't do it.

- When my husband is being negative and critical of me.

- My husband's history of two significant relapses, which he only confessed to when he was caught. This is such a huge roadblock for me in the trust area. I can forgive him for what has happened, but that does not mean I can forget it where trust is concerned. To be honest, I expect he will relapse again.

- My husband failing his first polygraph exam. I see it as evidence of his deeply entrenched habit of lying, even to himself.

- My husband's anger, contempt, arrogance, pride, and resentments, and continuing to live his life in secret.

- Several mentioned their partner's defensiveness as a problem. Here are some of their specific comments:

    - His defensiveness if I ask a question.

    - He wants everything in the relationship to be half my fault instead of taking responsibility for his acting out.

    - His defensiveness. I have always thought that because his addiction destroyed my trust, he should also be responsible for helping to restore it. I haven't yet felt that it is a priority for him.

- His lack of empathy for me.

- Him minimizing his acting out.

- His threatening divorce and saying he's not happy.

- Him putting work first.
- Him staying comfortable with the in-house separation arrangement; blaming me and wanting me to be the one to fix the relationship.
- The severity of my husband's acting-out behaviors.
- Society seems to think it is normal for men to act out.
- My spouse has ADHD and uses it as an excuse for problems we encounter.
- Knowing that he probably still lies to me but he believes he is protecting me.
- He is a noncommunicator. I would like reassurance (once in a while) that he is doing well with his therapy, that he does still love me, that he would never again consciously do anything that could destroy our marriage, our family, his reputation, or our financial future.
- Not doing homework given by his therapist and his sponsor.
- Going into denial and not owning his poor decisions.
- Spouse learning to deal with anger and blame.
- When things come up and I realize that he wasn't 100 percent honest when we started the process of recovery. Even though it's in the past, it makes me doubt how honest he has been in other things.
- He tends to avoid the tough subjects, so when something comes up and there is this big elephant in the room, so to speak, and he completely ignores it, I don't trust that he has made much progress.
- Hearing about his triggers.
- The bad choices he makes. For example, going to a woman hairdresser to get a haircut was not a good choice for him based on his past behavior.

WHAT WAS MOST BENEFICIAL TO RESTORING TRUST?
- Disclosure and polygraph (mentioned by several).

- My partner opening up and being honest about his addiction and how long it's been going on.

- Him communicating with me about his feelings.

- Intensive outpatient work with both of us.

- Polygraph testing of my spouse. But this process has just started with the formal disclosure process. I will not even consider physical intimacy until I can verify with a polygraph exam that he has not acted out for a year.

- My husband seems to be truthful in all things, even things that have no connection to the addiction. (Maybe he fears the polygraph exam!)

- Doing an evening devotional together.

- He is finally open about his struggle and how he is dealing with it.

- Not having to worry about going out in public and being humiliated by him constantly watching anyone who is in a skirt.

- Husband willing to have a strong Internet filter on his computer and parental controls on the TV.

- Relationship is different in that we are in the process of going through divorce. But I still have a general belief in the goodness of my former spouse.

- What has helped is him regularly seeing a competent therapist.

- We do recovery activities together every week, and that helps.

- Doing what was prescribed by our therapist + consistency = trust.

- Having access to passwords.

- Connecting with other women who've gone through this. These women have been voices of support though my journey.

- Knowing where he is. Him checking in with me from landlines— not cell phones.

- Seeing my husband's relentless pursuit of freedom and healing.

- The understanding my husband has of how much his sex addiction has hurt me and how negatively it has affected my life.

- Prayer.

- Praying together regularly.

- Him beginning to take responsibility for acting out rather than blaming external factors.

- A very powerful factor was him requesting information about how he could make amends to me.

- His willingness to be open with his schedule and what he is doing.

- My husband passed two polygraph exams, which proved to me he is not lying anymore. The fact that we can go back for more polygraph exams throughout our future to let me know if he is lying about anything.

- My husband and I have started talking quietly about the addiction, and he answers questions.

- My husband attends two twelve-step meetings regularly and is visibly altering certain negative behaviors.

- I see a difference in the level of rage he displays, and there has been no violence for some time.

- He practices rigorous honesty.

- When my husband has a peaceful, spiritual, and positive outlook on life. This usually happens as a result of him working the twelve-step program.

- Witnessing the beginnings of my husband's self-awareness with regard to his triggers, his pride, his fears, his entitlement, and his personal weaknesses (such as lying).

- My husband's sincere attempt to be a very good father to our sons, being a consistent and responsible provider for our family, and a kind and very generous friend and roommate.

- Emotionally focused couples therapy.

- Time and watching my spouse's actions, not just his words.

- The very first thing we did after I discovered his acting out was to make our separate bank accounts visible. Because everything had been separate since before we were married, I never knew where he spent money and how much. Now I can look at his accounts anytime I "need" to. If there is something that is questionable, I ask. He doesn't like it, but I ask.

- Accountability with money, accountability with time and his whereabouts.

- My husband's willingness to have a GPS tracking device on his phone and stay in contact with me when he is away.

- Listening to my hurts and not getting defensive.

- Admitting that what he did was wrong and apologizing.

- Getting rid of text messaging on his phone.

- Establishing set times for arriving home.

- When he takes initiative to share stresses (sexual or otherwise).

- His consistent contact with his sponsor.

- Him reaching out to his accountability partners and wanting to be involved with other men in recovery.

Partners Who Reported Significant Trust in the Relationship

Twenty-four percent of partners who responded to the survey reported that they had significant trust in their sex addict partners. Yet even with trust rebuilt, there are still factors that tended to erode that trust.

WHAT WAS LEAST BENEFICIAL TO RESTORING TRUST?

- For a time there was continued acting out that I found out about on my own. And to cover up the truth, my husband continued to lie to me, thinking he was getting away with his unacceptable behavior. With each event, the trust became less and less.

- When we don't communicate properly.

- When we are in a social setting with sexy women.

- The fact that he lied so much when I first discovered his acting out.

- My husband's statements that I can trust him.

- His continuing issues with lying about things unrelated to his sex addiction.

- In the beginning, the absence of other sex addicts sharing their success stories in public.

- Frequently hearing about slips and relapses from others who are in recovery, especially those who seem to be very serious about recovery.

- Listening to others. I know that sounds bad, but I can't listen to the hearsay of the other spouses or even my own mother when it comes to this. I have to be true to myself.

- What I heard from partners in some twelve-step meetings made me want to decrease the trust I had in him.

- My fear that he would not be trustworthy, open, and honest about working on his recovery.

- When he would check in with me and not disclose something he should have.

- When he would defend himself or get angry when he did something wrong.

- My partner's attitude.

- Clamming up and not talking to me about his past.

- Not keeping his promises.

- Him being arrogant.

- Him constantly criticizing political and religious leaders.

- My own horror at how low he went.

- Feeling guilty for forgiving him.

- The fact that other women he has acted out with are still around.

- Him taking so long to completely answer all my questions.

- My husband's habit of waiting until the next polygraph is near to tell me things he should have told me sooner.

- Accountability software. It has many flaws.

- Husband being impatient at first and saying I should "get over it."

- The fact that he still receives porn jokes from people on his email and won't delete them.

- Substance use.

- Arguments with my partner.

- When he is not willing to give up some behavior that makes me uncomfortable.

- Anytime my husband shows a lack of patience.

- Anytime my husband doesn't take responsibility for his own actions, no matter how minor the issue.

WHAT WAS MOST BENEFICIAL TO RESTORING TRUST?

For those who have reestablished significant trust in their partners, there were specific factors that helped them get there.

- Marriage counseling.

- Weekly check-ins between partners.

- Open communication about how I feel about the addiction and recovery.

- Attending twelve-step meetings for couples.

- My husband volunteering information about his struggles and how he chooses to handle them.

- Time.

- Working the Twelve Steps.

- Open and honest communication.

- Working on our relationship daily.

- Going to retreats together.

- Several mentioned polygraph exams. Here are some specific comments:

  - Polygraph exams are the most important ingredient coupled with sessions of therapy. I've come much further in the few years since he's been taking one yearly than when he wasn't.

  - Full disclosure with polygraph follow-up.

- Watching my husband work hard to get at, identify, and deal with his demons.

- Support, patience, and empathy from my husband.

- Seeing motivation and consistency in my husband's recovery activities.

- Praying together.

- Doing weekly exercises given by our therapist.

- Husband attending twelve-step meetings.

- Putting trust in my gut feelings. Had I listened to them in the past, things would have gone differently. They were right on the mark a decade ago, and I chose to tell myself, "Oh, that can't be true." But it was. So I listen to that voice inside me now.

- A growing relationship with God and then trusting to let go and let God work.

- It has helped that he checks in with me when he's on his way home from therapy or his twelve-step meetings or doing errands, even though I don't ask him to. I realize that deep down I need that reassurance.

- Understanding my part.

- My husband being willing to do anything it took to get help for himself and work on the root issues.

- My husband being consistent in the daily things he agreed to do.

- Him working on himself with a counselor. (Several partners in this group mentioned the sex addict getting counseling and therapy as being an important element in rebuilding trust.)

- Seeing his heart change.

- Slowly over time getting to know my husband as a different man, a changed man.

- Having our communication with each other change to be more positive and productive.

- Him being patient with me in allowing me to slowly move back toward him in an intimate way.

- Over the past three to five years, seeing God mold him into a totally different man.

- My husband finally grasping what rigorous honesty actually is. When he finally got to the point that he could tell me things that were hard to fess up to, no matter the consequences.

- Commitment to continually improving as individuals and having a partner who is as committed as I am.

- Learning to be relational.

- Learning to communicate functionally.

- I've learned to listen to my instinct, gut feeling, spirit—whatever one calls it. I do rest in knowing that God brought me through once and He will do it again if need be.

- So far all is well, but I'm not willing to trust words so easily. Instead I do acknowledge actions.

- Prayer.

- Communication tools.

- He has confessed times of temptation to me.

- He does not minimize what he did before.

- Him being able to ask for help.

- He calls often and lets me know where he is and what he is doing.

- He does not get upset when I question him and is willing to prove that he is saying the truth, and he does this in a calm manner.

- I have access to his email and cell phone accounts.

- His accountability for his time, money, and Internet use.

- His new relationship with God.

- His many behavioral changes.

- His sincere remorse, his kindness, and the love he gives me.

- Leading and supporting me gently without dominating me or making demands.

- Our renewed sexual relationship and his appreciation for me sexually.

- His patience and willingness to listen to me. His answering my questions. It works well for me to write them out for him to answer thoughtfully without emotions running high.

- The boundaries he has set and keeps.

- Confession (disclosure) to me and our children helps him with accountability and shows a change in his life.

- We are truly companions now and spend most of our time together working near each other, doing fun things, and going most places together. He has won my heart back.

- Taking care of myself.

- My husband's behavior. He is now walking the walk with obvious transparency and willingness to answer any question I have without hesitation or a negative attitude.

- Husband's medication appears to be helping with his impulse-control issues.

- My attitude. Regardless of what happens with him, I am just fine.

- Creating a culture of appreciation and disclosure in our relationship, putting the problem in perspective, compassion, understanding, commitment, and love.

- We have an agreement that I can ask any questions about the past or current activities.

- He voluntarily deleted his Facebook account.

- When he does not get angry or defensive when I ask questions about where he has been or question charges on credit cards or how he has spent money.

Partners Who Reported Complete Trust in the Relationship

This group of respondents was very small—only two participants said they fully trust their spouse. However, since full trust seems so elusive and because it is likely the goal of partners, what is shared by these two is nonetheless significant.

WHAT WAS LEAST BENEFICIAL TO RESTORING TRUST?

- Me "stuffing it" and not speaking it out loud.

- Thinking I could do it on my own. Forgetting to turn this entire thing over to God.

WHAT WAS MOST BENEFICIAL TO RESTORING TRUST?

- Seeing him go to meetings every week (which demonstrates his commitment to recovery). Him openly sharing about thought patterns that he identifies as contributors. Him taking the initiative to research movies before watching them. He confessed unprompted when he had a "slip-up."

- Learning to trust myself first. Speaking of my fear and suspicion in a healthy way to my husband. Working Steps One, Two, and Three of the Twelve Steps over and over in the beginning of recovery. Being gentle with myself, over and over again.

I hope this chapter has helped to expand your awareness of the possibility that trust can be restored in your relationship. Whether you are the wounded partner or the sex addict, you have a part to play in this process. While not easy or automatic, rebuilding trust is a goal worth pursuing. I have worked with numerous wounded partners who made it very clear at the beginning of therapy that they would never trust their spouse again. However, with hard work both individually and as a couple, couples can experience significant trust restoration in their relationship. Through persistence and hard work, trust can once again bloom in your relationship.

All but three of the twenty-six partners who reported either significant or full trust in the relationship have also experienced significant healing. The remaining three who reported significant trust experienced some healing. If sex addicts want trust to be restored in their relationship, they certainly need to be concerned with their partner's healing.

SURVEY SUMMARY

Twenty-six out of 103 survey respondents reported having regained significant or full trust in their partner. Another forty reported regaining some trust. Most important, one in five of the partners surveyed reported having made considerable progress in terms of both healing and trust.

For those wounded partners who have no trust in their sex-addicted partner, there are some common reasons:

- Nine survey participants cited inconsistency in the sex addict's recovery.

- Seven partners indicated a significant factor was the sex addict's continued lies and deceptions.

- Four reported that the attitude of the sex addict toward the partner (discounting wounded partner's needs, impatient with partner, or expecting partner to "get over it") was a factor, and three cited continued acting out as being reasons that there is no trust.

For partners who reported that some trust had been restored in their relationship, the factors that have had the most negative impact are these:

- Nine reported that it is the attitude toward the partner (discounting wounded partner's needs, impatient with partner, or expecting partner to "get over it").
- Four indicated inconsistency in the sex addict's recovery.
- Four mentioned continued lies and deception by the sex addict.
- Three pointed out their partner's continued acting out.

It is noteworthy that only six of the survey respondents in all the groups cited continued acting out as being a factor. Stopping all acting out will not automatically rebuild trust. For trust to be restored, sex addicts must also be consistent in all of their recovery efforts, stop all lying, and be committed to being part of the healing process with their wounded partner.

CHAPTER 18

WHAT ABOUT SEX?

While both parties will find this chapter useful, this chapter is more specifically addressed to the wounded partner.

Protect Yourself

What about your sexual relationship with your sex-addicted partner? The very first thing you need to do is to protect yourself. After discovering that your partner is a sex addict, you need to get tested for all sexually transmitted diseases. You need to do this even if you have gotten assurances from your partner that it is not necessary.

Prior to a clinical disclosure and a passed polygraph exam, you cannot be sure of the level of your risk. After disclosure and a polygraph to verify the disclosure, combined with a pattern of solid recovery and follow-up polygraph exams to ensure acting out has not recurred, you can feel safer being sexual with your spouse. But being assured of physical safety is not enough. You also need to feel safe emotionally. Working toward recovery with your partner results in enhanced communication between the two of you and greater emotional intimacy. Emotional intimacy is foundational for a healthy sexual relationship.

Your partner may pressure you to be sexual before you are ready or against your will. Some sex addicts tell their partner that they have to be sexual together to keep him or her from acting out. Do not give in to this pressure. If your partner cannot keep from acting out while you are asking for time to feel safe, what will he or she do on a business trip? And how will he or she be able to remain sexually sober if you are in poor health for an extended period of time and are unable to be sexual?

You cannot keep your partner from acting out, whether or not you are being sexual together. When you are feeling safer with your partner, you will be more ready to resume the sexual relationship. Until then, let your focus be on your own healing.

Sexual Anorexia

What about the cases where the sex addict does not want to be sexual with you? After the sexual acting out stops, it takes a while for the neurochemistry of the sex addict to readjust and settle down. What he or she has been getting from the addictive sexual behavior is a neurochemical response that is far in excess of that which comes from healthy sexual behavior in a committed relationship. That is not a result of a failing on the part of the wounded partner, but rather a function of getting addicted to the extreme neurochemical highs that come from the rush of acting out and all of its associated activities.

Much like drug addicts needing to learn to live without their drug's highs, sex addicts need time to adjust to normal neurochemical responses. When sex addicts completely eliminate all other sexual outlets, including sexual fantasy and masturbation, they can begin to build a healthy sexual appetite for their spouse.

There may also be a subconscious belief on the part of the sex addict that the solution to sex addiction is to stop having sex. He or she may swing from sexual acting out to sexual anorexia—a loss of interest in or "appetite for" emotionally intimate sexual interaction. Often this knee-jerk reaction is self-correcting as time passes.

Intimacy vs. Intensity

Sex addiction is an intimacy disorder. While is it natural for people to have a desire for intimacy, sex addicts prior to recovery do not know how to achieve intimacy. Instead, they substitute intensity for intimacy. Their sexual acting out focused on intensity, and the escalated neurochemical response it created was part of that dynamic. During active sex addiction, even sex with a spouse is often focused on intensity, with the sex addict pressuring his or her partner to do things to add excitement to their sex life.

It is true that sex in a committed relationship can be very intense. But the goal should not be intensity, but rather intimacy. It is healthiest when intensity is a byproduct of intimate sexual interaction. When intensity results, be happy for it. But also recognize that intimacy is also achieved, which is the ultimate goal in any marriage or committed relationship.

In resuming a sexual relationship, you will want to know that when you are with your sex-addicted partner, he or she is completely with you. You want to know that your partner is present with you and not reliving an old acting-out event or a fantasy. One of the best ways to know that he or she is with you is to look into his or her eyes. If you can see your partner's eyes while you are being sexual, you can know whether your partner is with you mentally and emotionally or if he or she has zoned out.

Let your sexual relationship focus on being tender and loving toward one another. When these elements are present, they are typically evident well before a couple is engaged in sexuality. And do not be afraid to stop if you are not feeling safe. Your partner may not be at a place where he or she can accept that, but your continued emotional safety is paramount for your sexual relationship to resume in a healthy way.

Strive to redefine what sexuality is between the two of you. Avoid measuring it against whether either or both of you have an orgasm. Remove the requirement of intercourse as being the measure of whether or not you are sexual. You and your partner may be very sexual together without intercourse and find that the time is still deeply fulfilling for both of you.

Professional Help

While it is normal for couples in recovery to want to move toward healthy sex as soon as possible, this may be one of the last areas to improve. As natural as sex should be, when trying to get past an unhealthy sexual history, some couples find they can benefit from the help of a sex therapist. I would recommend this not take place in the Survival phase of recovery, but in the Stability phase or later. If you use a sex therapist, be sure to use one who understands sex addiction. Sex therapists without expertise in dealing with sex addiction may recommend things that would be harmful to the recovery of both the sex addict and his or her partner.

CHAPTER 19

SURVEY RESULTS: ADDITIONAL COMMENTS FROM PARTNERS

Besides responding to specific questions, those who completed the sex addict partner survey were given the option of adding any additional comments they wanted to make. Many took positive advantage of this opportunity to share their thoughts and feelings about their experiences with the sex addict in their life, the recovery process, and the status of their relationship.

One comment repeated by multiple respondents was their gratitude at receiving the survey and being asked about their journey. Several said that completing the survey helped them to process some of their feelings and make further sense of their experiences. With that in mind, I am reminded of the value of processing feelings by writing in a journal. While only a few partners mentioned the value of journaling, many more of the couples I have worked with have spoken about the healing quality of journaling.

The following are additional comments from the survey participants:

- Our relationship is deeper than it ever would have been if we hadn't gone through recovery together.

- I was sad that after thirty-four years of marriage I had to file for divorce, but I cannot do any more to save this relationship when he can't control his choices.

- Face-to-face support proved to accelerate the healing process for me. The phone support was good, but "seeing" the other person showing empathy or concern or care was like a healing balm.

- This is the hardest journey I have had to travel, because the person I have been married to has continued to live in denial of his addiction. Because of this, he continues to blame me and our relationship for his issues. It takes a while to see this as part of his sickness and for me to be able to move away from it. As I look back at my journey, I know many times I became out of control with my anger, hurt, and pain, and that did not help recovery for myself. I have to forgive myself for those times and move forward with a better ability to control my emotions in order to be a better representation of the person I am. I take a step every day to reclaim my life and my choices as my spouse seems to continue to choose sickness.

- I have learned a tremendous amount of information about addiction and what the addict goes through. Although I will not accept this information as an excuse for his unacceptable behavior, it allows me to better understand his struggles. I have also learned a great deal of information about what partners go through. This has helped give me permission to grieve and feel my own pain. I have set clear boundaries with my husband and will keep them throughout our marriage. He knows how serious I am about this because I've set boundaries along the way, and when he crossed them I stood strong and followed through on my word. I feel that probably the most important thing the partner must do is be true to self no matter how much you stand in place and claim your love for your partner. I love my husband very much, and that is the reason we are still together. But I have also set boundaries and kept them. He respects me that much more for keeping them. I continue to learn and nurture myself, my husband, and our coupleship in recovery. This is a lifestyle for us, not a short-time cure.

- The sex addict needs to be honest. Finding out I was in a relationship with a sex addict was hard, but by working the Twelve Steps we are a stronger couple. We have better communication skills. The partner needs to look inside herself. Is she codependent? Is she enabling? I have been codependent forever and never dealt with my own issues. By his sex addiction coming to light, I began to heal and work on myself.

- Looking at pornography is a betrayal, and society fosters the acceptance of this betrayal by shrugging its shoulders with the attitude that "it's just what guys do." I think that one of the hardest things to deal with is knowing that most people view pornography this way. Or they feel that the woman must just not be "giving it up" enough, and now both the shame and the blame are passed on to the victim. There are billboards that advertise drug and alcohol addiction counseling services, as well as commercials on television and radio. It would be amazing if counseling for sex addiction would be advertised as well. I think that then a person with a partner who has a sex addiction would feel less isolated, as well as more courageous about seeking help.

- Do not think that there is a quick or permanent fix. Do not think that because one day is good, the next will be good. Do not think that because one day is bad, the next will be bad. Acknowledge the past and the pain, but live in the present.

- I am a true believer in intensive outpatient therapy for couples, combined with a polygraph exam. My husband never would have freely admitted to or come clean regarding what he had done.

- I see too few sex addiction therapists educating addicts about how to be supportive of and empathetic to their spouses. Addicts must understand that they cannot expect praise or validation from their partner, especially in the first several months. They must seek support from other men, as well as through therapy. If his therapist guides him, as the injuring partner, in supporting her, then she will usually be able to be supportive of him sooner. But if he cannot learn to empathize, it may take forty years, but she will eventually grow cold and bitter and all hope for the marriage will be lost.

- I am so thankful that my husband sought help for himself and our marriage. I am glad he found our therapist. The help we have received from him has been such a blessing. I think the greatest factor in helping us heal is the weekly recovery activities we do together. I love seeing the brokenness and authenticity of my husband during our time of prayer and sharing. I love having my trust bucket filled.

- I wish there were more places that the partner could go when the addict won't get help. Too many spouses play the "victim card" or the "oh, poor me card," and they use it to a degree that causes them to never heal. I can't do that! Accept things and move on, either with or without your addict spouse, but make a stance and stick to it and stop being the victim.

- If my husband would quit acting out and become sober, I would feel better about our chances for staying together. He says he wants to stay married, but it would help if he would agree to continue his therapy.

- I just want to say again how important the polygraph exam is in this process. I've been in a relationship with a sex addict for over twenty years. He obviously is a good liar, so before the polygraph exam I was constantly trying to verify what he told me. I was looking outside if he told me it was raining. He would lie about everything! Whoever said you can't love someone if you don't trust them is wrong. You can, but it makes life extremely hard. I have always had hope, but it definitely was dwindling fast. I was at a point where I didn't want to be with him anymore, and I was picturing what it would take to leave him. The polygraph exam was the only change we added (and a good therapist) to his recovery process. When he passed, I could trust my time with him again—no more detective work. From that time forward I could breathe. I'll always be scarred by our past, but we're moving forward again. I don't know how many more years I'll need him to take a polygraph exam, but for now, I know I need him to continue to be willing to do this annually.

- I feel that the biggest thing that helped me was the therapy in our intensive outpatient treatment. You are really not sure if you are sane by the time you get to the stage I was at. It helps to be able to totally open up with someone who is trained in this problem. It helped me to be able to see my husband as someone who was not a bad person, but a very sick person. I was convinced I could never get to that place. It helped me to think through how to get my life back even if my husband didn't recover.

- Before my intensive outpatient treatment, I had never encountered anyone, even my close friend, who would encourage me to move forward. I read what someone had written about the sex addiction problem. It is like standing in the driveway behind your husband's car. He backs up and runs over you. He hits his head on the dash when the car impacts you. On his forehead there is a bleeding cut. Neighbors come from everywhere to help him. The medics come and make a big fuss over him and he gets the best of medical care. Meanwhile, they have forgotten that the wife is still under the car.

- I would love for someone to have a magical wand to make it all go away. More follow-up care would be appreciated, or some kind of group that can meet via an Internet phone call.

- The wives read all sorts of material in sex addiction books including books for partners about "what it means to be male." In the books for the male sex addict there is very little, if any, information for him about "what it means to be female." He does understand that this has hurt me, but really does not have any understanding as to the depth of this pain and all the emotions that go with that. He also equates forgiveness with trust and does not understand that these do not go hand in hand. More information for the male addict about his wife and her journey would be a huge benefit to them both.

- I highly recommend that both parties engage in some form of personal therapy.

- Safety, time, and support, combined with a growing relationship with the Lord, overcome and heal most anything.

- I wish there were more resources available to sex addicts and partners down here in Australia. There needs to be more focus on PTSD symptoms. It is real! The excruciating pain is indescribable. I don't think the world quite gets this. Most people misattribute everything as being a normal relationship breakup, or they blame the victim. The blaming has retraumatized me. There needs to be more focused information for mothers of sex addicts. It would be very beneficial to help them cope, too. Often they can get stuck in denial. A video specifically for mothers would be good.

- From the beginning of this nightmare, I have told my husband that I need him to talk to me, to tell me the whole sordid story, so I can stop imagining my own scenarios. I need to know everything so I can put it away and move forward. It is so painful for him to talk to me about it, even after my "knowing" for over two years. I don't know if he will ever tell me all of it. I know I will never be such a Pollyanna again, but he is still my true love and my best friend. I want to look at all of it, then set it aside and move forward.

- Contact with him puts me on an emotional roller coaster. One day he wants to be restored with his family, the next day he doesn't. Each time he turns away again, my heart moves further away from him, and I move toward thinking that divorce sounds like a vacation.

• My heart goes out to those involved in this very devastating illness. It is difficult to understand how strong the desire can be for something so senseless that someone would risk everything they have financially, emotionally, and spiritually. There are scars that never fully heal, I'm afraid.

• Partners of sex addicts are primarily left to heal on our own. We must search and find anything or anyone who is "safe" to talk to. To find out if they are our "safe" people, we have to put our story out there and take the chance of being judged, blamed, or rejected. Our world has been turned upside down and it has basically left me with two choices, neither of which are good. I can stay with my sex-addicted spouse and live with the pain of infidelity for the rest of my life, or leave my marriage and break apart my entire family because of his sex addiction. It leaves spouses with few good options. Many spouses who want to leave the marriage do not have jobs (like me) to support themselves. I stayed home to raise our children and my husband didn't want me to work after they were raised, so I am dependent solely on him financially. Economic insecurity and healthcare concerns then become traumatizing. There is also the burden of being the one to break up the family and dealing with their devastation if I choose divorce. This is very traumatizing for a woman, especially an older woman like me. I believed I would grow old with my husband, who I thought was faithful to me.

• Because his addiction has gone on for so long in our marriage, I know it will take some time to restore the trust. My husband is currently in between jobs. I would value the opportunity to be engaged in counseling that really works. However, without the aid of health insurance, we are limited. This is why I would welcome some sort of couples retreat or group to help us with our struggles for the time being. For now I would have to say we are hanging on with hope and a prayer.

- Sex addiction is such a complicated problem that there is no way we would have found our way out of the maze without intense professional help. We tried—not just tried, but almost died trying. It is just not covered in any part of life's training.

- Videos we have watched about recovery have been very helpful.

- There is such a lack of support for partners. The disclosure has been so traumatic for me. There are a lot of groups to help support my husband. I was even supposed to be part of his support. But how can I be supportive for him when I have just been traumatized? My entire married life has been one lie after another. It has been eighteen months and I have been to counselors on a weekly basis for about eight of those months, but none of them seem to understand. I have no control. I even went through a period of hitting myself because it was the only "thing" I could do. My husband refuses to participate in any recovery programs, even if it is only to make me feel better. He says he isn't cheating on me anymore, so he thinks that should be good enough. He has little patience with me.

- Ever since I found out about his acting out it has been an emotional roller coaster, with times when I could've sworn I was going crazy. I have heard from other women that they all went through similar experiences. We are not crazy; our lives as we knew them were shattered. When I learned to look at his addiction for what it is—a sickness—and not take it as an intentional act to hurt me, I was able to manage the anger better.

- It is a difficult journey, but having God as our focus is changing everything!

- I don't know where this is going. It would be helpful to have more of a picture of what long-term recovery looks like.

- I love him. I meant my wedding vows even though he said he did not mean his. If he wants a marriage partner, he needs to act like he wants one. I cannot be the overseer of his recovery or his accountability partner. It depends on whether he just wants a roommate or a wife—with all of the nuances of a relationship that entails. The thing that amazes me is that before I met my husband I was in a three-year relationship with someone I knew was a sex addict. I did not know it immediately, but when I found out I left the relationship. I was attracted to my husband for many reasons, but I thought he was a safe harbor after the previous relationship. They were absolutely different in their sexual behavior. I have never been as shocked as when I found out my husband was a sex addict too. I'm amazed at the amount of hiding he had to do. He and I both have been in Narcotics Anonymous for twenty-three years, so I was not ignorant about addiction, at least where drugs are concerned. I felt the disease of sex addiction had sneaked up from behind and bitten me.

• There is only some trust because there is only some recovery. The process is painful, and therefore it is easy for the addict to decide that enough is enough and that this is good enough. It is sad because it could be so much better. However, although it took me a while to get healthy, I can continue to work on myself and I am doing so. I expect to be in a better state as I work the Twelve Steps more and more.

• I would so appreciate the opportunity to attend counseling or purchase resources at a reduced rate. I was married thirty-five years and a stay-at-home mom with four kids. It has truly been devastating.

• I think that the intensive program we attended is the best there is out there, but as I have learned, you can lead a horse to water but you can't make it drink. I want to say that I was so very excited to work through the steps and use the tools that our therapist gave us at our Intensive. I also want to say that I will never forget the feeling I had when I realized that my husband had no intention of following through with it and refused to submit himself to the things that were outlined for him to do to obtain his freedom and rebuild our marriage. My heart was literally pounding inside my chest, and my hopes were dashed one more time. I gave it two more years, but now I have decided to move on. May the couples who seek help in the future both come with total surrender and willingness to do what it takes to heal their marriages and lives.

• I don't believe a couple can be successful in overcoming the devastation caused by sex addiction without a strong commitment to God. If the addicted partner is not willing to turn his or her life over to God and beg for help, he or she will not be able to defeat the beast. Only God can give the strength and comfort that both partners need. God is first, and then a strong support system and good resources for information are necessary.

• Despite love and commitment, when boundaries are set and breached repeatedly, partners find themselves in a position to move out of the relationship to prevent the cycle from continuing. Trust and intimacy can be shattered to the point of no return. Given a pattern of lying and not practicing safe sex, a spouse risks her physical and emotional well-being by reengaging. It would take a daily polygraph to not feel at risk.

• It was a long, difficult, and painful journey, but I am so thankful to God for the change He has made in my life as well as my husband's life. We both changed, and we got to know each other all over again. There was no way I wanted to stay married to the man he was, and God answered my prayer. God gave us a new life together, and now we've been married twenty-five years.

• I wish the pain would end.

• It takes two!

• We wouldn't be where we are today without the Lord, and I know that He worked through our therapist. I believe the work that we did saved our marriage.

• My husband and I have been in recovery for one year and four months. He has been able to stay sober. A big part of the credit for our recovery goes to the methods used by our therapist. We pretty much follow his recommendations, which include regular polygraphs. I believe that this is an integral component in our recovery. It helps my husband stay sober and it helps me to detach from his recovery. For me, working on my recovery through my twelve-step fellowship has been incredible. I have made friends from all over the United States and I have strengthened my relationship with my higher power. I feel that I am a much stronger and more spiritual person because of my recovery.

• My husband and I have been separated now for nearly three months. He stayed at home on the West Coast and I went 3,000 miles away to the East Coast to stay with family. We took this time in order to be able to work on our own individual recoveries without having to also manage our day-to-day relationship at the same time. This separation was supported by both my individual counselor and his therapist who also sees us together. I will be returning home in one month. I know that I have made progress in my own recovery because I never would have felt comfortable being gone this long. Before recovery I hated even going to the store for a few hours because I knew what would be going on at home. I do not trust that my husband is not acting out while we are separated now, but at the same time I am able to let go of that distrust and do what I need to do for my own healing. I know I have to find my own path, whatever that is, regardless of whether or not he is acting out. This shows me that I have made significant progress in the year working my twelve-step program. I have no idea what it will be like when I return home. I have no idea how I will feel or what I will decide. I know that what I want is a renewed and honest relationship with my husband. I don't know if that's possible. I want to know that I have a final and truthful disclosure so that I can finally put the past to rest and let go of my hypervigilance in waiting for another bomb to drop. I would like my husband to take a polygraph test in order to finally get the honest truth and have it verified that there is nothing left to disclose. Until then, there will be zero trust, unfortunately.

• I think one major huge gap that goes unaddressed or underresponded to is the risk of STDs like HIV and AIDS. I do not think women should be encouraged to resume sexual relations so soon. Their life is at stake. I have not found this issue to be addressed honestly or seriously. Women are made to feel bad that there is something wrong with them for not resuming sexual contact, as if she is using this against her husband instead of as a valid protection of herself.

• I am in the process of accepting that my husband has years of work to do on himself before I will consider trusting him with the most sacred part of my heart. After months of prayer, Christ has placed that on my heart. I live day to day, and sometimes week to week, but at this point it is hard to make any long-term future plans with my husband.

• If there is a separation, do not allow the husband to move back in until the Twelve Steps have been completed with a sponsor. Use the leverage of separation to see that work is done while there is motivation. The entire addiction experience, especially sex addiction, comes with an enormous spiritual battle. It has been hand-to-hand combat with the enemy for our entire marriage, and he does not want to let go. Test the addict for personality disorders in case there are multiple layers of problems. My husband is stuck in shame and is addicted to only feeling shame because it has gone on literally his whole life. Regular counseling just keeps him stuck as a victim. Match up survivor couples with newly hurting couples to increase both couples' recovery.

• Three and a half years after discovering my husband's addiction, we have moved past the worries of sex addiction, triggers, and slips and are now following a more spiritual path of self-improvement. I know this is no doubt due to our therapist's skill and care in handling my husband's full disclosure to me, as well as his caring concern for my well-being and his accessibility and nonjudgmental attitude. This was a very delicate situation, and in hindsight after reading dozens of books on sex addiction, I realize how important it was for our therapist to guide us through disclosure in an effort not to retraumatize me.

- I journaled this morning and had additional things come up that I wanted to say: Recovery is much harder than living in the addiction cycle. I still see acting-out behavior—irritability, drinking, yelling, blaming, and defensiveness—but now he is addicted to sports, work, travel, and food. The addict needs to view the partner as a trauma victim. In our situation, the *co-addict* term gets used as a means of blame and as an excuse for the addict to stay stuck as a victim. Few counselors are hard on the addict. The addict can stay stuck and continue the addiction cycle in the counseling office, making every story into the addict being a victim and never moving forward.

- It is very important for the partner to have a therapist who understands both addiction and trauma. Simply labeling someone as a co-sex addict is disempowering.

- I have found it nearly impossible to have a significant recovery apart from my spouse having ongoing recovery. Much of the literature would call me codependent, telling me that I should have no problem recovering by concentrating on myself. Unfortunately, I have a hard time recovering when I'm always wondering when the other shoe will drop and wondering how bad it will be the next time it does. Difficult decisions must be made when small children must be considered.

- I've learned that I play a role in all of this. I've learned that drilling or even complaining does not help. Saying clearly what I want once and dropping it, then allowing him to choose whether or not he does it, works. Not threatening to leave him works, too. Telling him, "I'm not leaving you. I love you, but this particular behavior (whatever it is) is unacceptable," and then acting as though nothing is wrong works. He tries to please me when I clearly state what I want without nagging and complaining and preaching. This has been my most beneficial tool since my crisis.

- I feel my situation is unique, since we are not married. However, I feel blessed to have had the opportunity to know about and begin to understand this addiction early in our relationship. We are building a future based on honesty. That is everything! We know our challenges with this addiction and have the tools to overcome it and grow through it. Remaining together is not based on a long-term marriage or children, as is the case for so many. I feel we have the freedom to stay together and stand against this addiction together. That takes so many obstacles out of our path and allows the focus to be about us individually and as a couple.

- Because of my health crisis, I have no choice but to focus on my health and well-being. Sadly, it took such an incident for me to realize the damage the stress and frustration of this situation has caused me. I have committed to working on restoring my strength and developing strategies that will be of help to me regardless of the future of the relationship.

- I believe that the sex addict is treated in a way that he is able to heal but the partner is left to her own luck.

- I think it is also important to let my husband know that his efforts are appreciated and that I am really proud of him. I feel the fact that he went to therapy to save our marriage was the best gift he could give me. We attended a couples retreat, and that was the best experience for both of us.

- I wish I could help him understand that I genuinely do want the truth always. I prefer truth to lies. I do know it's hard for him to tell me the truth, but I need it and I want it and I deserve it. He can trust me to tell the truth about what I need from him.

- This has been the greatest hardship of my life. I feel like I have barely survived the last three years. It has been extremely hard. He knew exactly what I thought of affairs and sexual behavior, and he knew I thought if one partner were to decide to do it, they should tell the other and allow for divorce. Instead, he did it and kept it a secret from me. He knew that it would be more than I could handle. I discovered his acting out in 2008. Then I lost my job of thirty-one years as an RN at a hospital because they closed my department in

2009. My unemployment has caused us great financial stress, but it was for the best, as I do not believe I could have worked during the time when I found out.

- It continues to amaze me on a daily basis now how incredibly destructive deviant sexual behavior can be. Maybe I've become oversensitive, but not a day goes by without me seeing some article in the paper or on television. Reminders are everywhere. Getting beyond them is a daily challenge.

- It seems as though few marriages survive sex addiction. My devotion to my children and to the person my husband is when he's not acting out kept me in the relationship. Time and the work we've both done on ourselves have made the last four years so much better than the first six. I don't want to sound like a gold digger, but both of us knowing that in our country ten years of marriage is the point where I would be eligible for one-half of my husband's pension if we were to divorce takes another level of pressure off me.

- It has been eighteen months since our first visit with our therapist. We have almost no sex life at all now. Sex addiction is such a horrible addiction because it is impossible to have any kind of normal sex life when sex is the very thing you are supposed to be abstaining from. What is normal, anyway? At this point I think I preferred the fake marriage we had for fifteen years because at least we had a sex life. I am slowly adapting and learning to live in a sexless marriage, and it isn't that bad.

- In my view, my husband just changing his actions, going to meetings, and the like doesn't change anything. Being a witness to my husband's heart being changed by Jesus Christ—this is true change. And faith that the Lord will not only heal my husband, but also heal me is what is getting me through.

- I appreciate all our therapist did to try to help our situation and our relationship. I am sad that my husband has been resistant to any help that has been offered to him.

- The information I am learning from phone therapy about personal empowerment and healthy detachment seems the most helpful so far.

- Hearing about the threats he experienced to his sobriety was incredibly painful at first, but was helpful in the long run when I acknowledge that he is being honest.

- I am proud of my husband's accomplishments for himself in recovery. Sometimes I wonder if he will be in recovery forever and whether it will ever feel like a truly trusting relationship to me.

- Healing and reconciliation are much more difficult than I realized. I still have very little to no hope that I will be able to trust my husband again. I have a hard time believing that he isn't going to continue the same cycle over and over again. I need this to be over. I need the addict to recover.

- I just wish we had more time for my husband to understand the devastating magnitude of what his acting out has done to myself, our boys, and also our extended family. I know I need as much support as possible because my husband is very good at dismissing my feelings and opinions. I hope there will be more men of integrity, and I hope my husband will be one of them.

- I have been married twenty-one years. I knew something was wrong, but my husband always said it was me being a bitch. He was not engaged with me as a husband or with my children as a father. He bad-mouthed me to others for most of our marriage and blamed me completely for everything. It all came to light one year ago with the discovery of his addiction, and all of a sudden everything made perfect sense. The worst part is that it really makes no sense at all! Pornography is completely senseless!

- Even though it was so long ago, I still feel I am healing. I have had some successful, healthy relationships with men, but it took five or six years to be in a place where I was open to trusting someone. Also, going back to my family of origin helped. I realized I had issues that I hadn't resolved with both parents, so with time there has been healing there as well.

- I wish there was more help for partners of sex addicts. Here in England there is nothing.

- I think different approaches to different people should be used. For instance, I think therapists should communicate in a sterner and more direct fashion with those with "difficult" personalities. The polygraph is a genius idea and helped greatly in my healing!

- There are awesome resources out there for addicts and spouses. Everyone is different; everyone's personality, maturity, and even spiritual maturity is different. However, I believe there are resources for everyone. We just have to search for them. If I could say one thing to the addicts, it is that diligence and sensitivity to the hurt partner go a long way.

CHAPTER 20

WHEN IS IT TIME TO MOVE ON?

Felix's Story

Felix is a good man. This was not just his self-evaluation; it was also that of Connie, his wife of twenty-seven years. He entered recovery twelve years ago. During those years he had experienced what he considered a slip about every three months. Each time, he convinced Connie to take another chance on him as he recommitted to making recovery a higher priority.

Felix always considered himself a bit shy. He had not dated much as a teenager. His wife was the first person he had ever kissed. He

WHEN IS IT TIME TO MOVE ON?

kept his various problematic sexual behaviors carefully hidden from her. Every two or three days, Felix would log in to a pornography site where he was a member to watch the latest videos. His favorite videos were those categorized as "barely legal"—videos of teenage girls who were at least 18 years old but appeared to be younger. Next, he would spend some time in adult chat rooms, again looking for older teenage girls willing to talk dirty to him. Felix found it easier to speak to teens.

On one occasion Felix was intrigued by an instant message from a girl who said, "I'm 15 but I look like I'm 25." He carried on a conversation with her over a period of six weeks. Several times she invited him to meet her in person, but at first he declined. Eventually he agreed to meet her at a shopping center, and was arrested when he stepped into the store. The girl was actually a federal agent posing as a juvenile to try to apprehend child predators who prey on unsuspecting children. Felix is now serving a sentence in a federal prison for solicitation of a minor and upon his release will be a registered sex offender.

There are times during the active addiction—and even in recovery—when spouses or partners wonder if it is time to end the relationship. This may not be a comfortable subject, but its consideration deserves attention.

It is tragic that many marriages are destroyed because of sex addiction. However, the discovery of problematic sexual behavior does not have to be the end of a relationship—even if that activity has involved other people and perhaps many other people. As I have noted throughout, if the sex addict is willing to get help and address the problematic sexual behavior, the relationship not only can be saved but can thrive in recovery.

Some individuals have the mistaken belief that if their spouse has been unfaithful, they must get a divorce. Not only is the unfaithfulness itself devastating, but spouses believe the acting out will occur again and again. Rather than look for a way out, couples can look for a way to stay in their relationship and put the pieces back together. It is possible for marriages rocked by sex addiction to be restored—if the addict is willing to do whatever it takes to get free from problematic sexual behavior and the partner is willing to go through the difficult process of healing and trauma resolution, and if they work together through the process of restoring trust.

Addictions often develop over a lifetime. They are behaviors reinforced by years of acting out and powerful neurochemical influences. Recovery may involve a series of starts and stops, and remissions followed by relapses. Rather than a steady uphill progression, it is more like a roller coaster with ups and downs, yet all the time moving forward.

If an individual is committed to a program of recovery, even if he or she continues to have setbacks, there is reason to hope that he or she will be able to get free from all compulsive behavior and live the rest of his or her life in sexual integrity. Do not lose hope!

When the Sex Addict Refuses Help

What about relationships where sex addicts are not willing to get help? If your partner admits to having difficulty with problematic sexual behavior but refuses to address that problem, it is time to consider ending the relationship.

When a partner sets this boundary and requires that the addict seek help, and the addict is convinced of the seriousness of the partner, he or she may realize the only choice left for saving the relationship is to get help with the addiction. I have had numerous cases where divorce papers had been filed, attorneys were retained, and couples were on their way to establishing separate lives, only to have the legal proceedings stopped when the sex addict decides to get help. This is not to suggest that threats of divorce or abandonment should be used to manipulate sex addicts into recovery. When a spouse reaches the point where he or she is getting ready to end the relationship, that decision may be enough to persuade the sex addict to seek immediate help.

Often sex addicts will come to their senses and do everything possible to save the relationship when they realize that their spouse is ready to end it. If the shock of the partner saying the relationship is over gets an addict into recovery, then he or she can be grateful that something was stronger than the power of addiction, and that was coming face-to-face with the loss of the relationship.

What about the cases where addicts continue to slip or relapse? How do you respond if they are not able to stay sexually sober? This may also be the time to consider ending the relationship. If that happens, recognize that it is the addict's decision to put addiction ahead of the relationship that resulted in forfeiture of the relationship.

No one works recovery perfectly. Unfortunately, many addicts have slips and relapses that punctuate their recovery. A single failure in recovery or even a couple of failures should not automatically bring an end to the relationship. If actions are taken to rectify the situation and restore solid recovery routines, the relationship may be salvaged.

But if the sex addict is not willing to do the work of recovery even after repeated opportunities to get help, it may be time to take steps to end the relationship and move on. Moving on may mean leaving your spouse trapped in his or her addiction. If this is the place you find yourself in, and you have given your partner repeated chances to get into recovery but he or she has refused or continues to act out, then you may feel that he or she has chosen the addiction over you. Ending the relationship is a difficult decision—one that you should make only after much soul-searching and consultation with professionals and trusted friends. Life without your partner will be challenging and perhaps painful, but ask yourself, what will the pain be like if you remain in the relationship and your partner's acting out is unending?

The Relationship Is Over. What Went Wrong?

In some cases, the relationship was over before the partner knew the extent of her or his spouse's addiction. Or maybe the sex addict announced that he or she had found someone who "really knows how to love me" and walked away from the relationship without trying to save it. Abrupt endings are devastating and leave lasting wounds.

Some sexually addicted individuals never get into recovery. In spite of the efforts of their partners, they continue to resist all offers of recovery. Their partners set boundaries, give ultimatums, make impassioned pleas, and otherwise beg their partners to get into recovery and give the relationship a chance. However, they are powerless over their partners' addictions and cannot bring them to recovery. In other cases, addicts continue to suffer slips and relapses. They make promises to stop their destructive behavior and even make some attempt to do the work of recovery, but it never sticks. After a few sessions of therapy and a few twelve-step meetings, they declare themselves "cured" and stop all recovery actions. The repeated relapses finally bring partners to the point of saying, "Enough!"

There are other relationships where the husband and the wife both get into recovery, but the relationship still does not work. For some, there was too great an imbalance in recovery; that is, one partner was well ahead of the other and the other never caught up. In others, even though recovery appears to be going well for both, they cannot make the relationship work.

Sometimes the wounds of deceit are too deep to heal. In some cases, one or both partners are unable to move to a place of acceptance as a prelude to forgiveness so that healing can begin. There are some spouses who have had so much trauma throughout life that they cannot cope with the additional trauma that was caused by the sex addict's active addiction. There are some recovering sex addicts who are so prideful in their recovery and their newfound sexual sobriety that they live in arrogance (even though humility—the opposite of arrogance—is one of the fundamental principles of healthy recovery) and insist that they are in the right and their partner is wrong. It really does not matter what finally happened, because the relationship is over. Wishing, hoping, crying, and pleading will not restore that which has been severed.

If I am describing your plight, if your relationship has ended, I have a few suggestions for you about your future. First, do not begin dating until you have continued further in your own recovery journey. You need time to make sense of your feelings and concentrate on yourself. No rebound relationship will provide the nurturing you now need. If you are dating currently, you would be well advised to stop immediately. You deserve to have time to take care of yourself, and this needs to be your priority. Life is not going to pass you by while you are concentrating on getting the support and healing that you need.

If you are not in therapy at present, I encourage you to start therapy immediately. If you have unresolved family-of-origin issues and/or childhood wounds, it is important to take the time and make the space to work on them. If you have trauma related to your ex-partner's sex addiction and/or other past experiences, this would also be a good time to consider finding an Eye Movement Desensitization and Reprocessing (EMDR) therapist who can help you address this.

It is especially important that you get professional help to determine what you got from the relationship with your former partner. You may be able to see some similarities between your former partner and other people with whom you have had previous relationships. Some individuals are candid and insightful enough to admit that they seem to always end up with someone who is an addict or someone who is abusive to them. Addicts are frequently charming, persuasive, and very focused on the person who is the object of their affection. If you have chosen an addict of any variety in any of your previous relationships, this would be a good time to ask yourself, "What do I need to do to heal, and to quit living out the same traumatic relationship patterns over and over again?"

If this describes you, you alone can change the next chapter of your life. You are the author of your own future. No matter how long you have let others tell you how to live your life, you are now free to assume control of the events in your life. You deserve a healthy relationship. Do not settle for less.

This would also be a good time for you to cement relationships with other men or women who are healing from relationships that have damaged their self-esteem. Twelve-step programs are important sources of support for individuals who have found themselves alone after the end of a relationship with a sex addict. But a word of caution: Be careful that you do not use twelve-step meeting rooms as a hunting ground for a new partner. Focus on your healing. Do your step work. Postpone the search for a new partner until you have experienced significant healing.

CHAPTER 21

CLOSING MESSAGE

Recovery Is an Adventure

I tell my clients that in the course of their recovery journey they will be able to look at themselves in the mirror and say, "You are a good person," and know from the bottom of their hearts that those words are true. The negative self-talk that has plagued them since childhood will gradually end and be replaced with self-caring, healing words. I believe recovery can truly become an adventure. In the end, recovering sex addicts and their partners—whether their relationship continues or does not—can have a much fuller, richer, more meaningful life than if they had not had compulsive behaviors to conquer.

Sex addiction recovery can be a wonderful adventure of discovery. As with many adventures, recovering from sex addiction continues throughout life. Sex addicts never get to the point where all of their recovery work is done. They continue to find new challenges to face and additional parts of their character upon which to focus. Yet as long as they are living free from destructive behavior, their active addiction is behind them. Their journey of freedom continues and never has to stop.

As you continue through the many tasks of recovery, you will find challenges and numerous blessings. As you and your partner take this journey, you will have the opportunity to work on yourselves in ways that would have escaped your notice if it were not for addiction and then for recovery.

In the Big Book of Alcoholics Anonymous,[40] in the section referred to as "the promises," it states that there will come a time when a person will "not regret the past nor wish to shut the door on it." While this may seem unattainable, it becomes reality for many. Perhaps it is more fully realized when a couple takes the recovery journey together.

Certainly there are hurts and pain from the past that bring excruciating grief. There are things that recovering addicts deeply regret. That regret is shared by their partners. Addiction wounds both the addicted and those who love them. It is a vicious circle that can only be severed by making a commitment to do the work necessary to end all compulsive behavior one day at a time, forever.

The presence of sex addiction in a relationship does not mean that a relationship must come to an end. Nor does it mean that happiness must end. If both the addict and the partner are willing to address the addiction and work on their individual recoveries and recovery as a couple, there is every reason to hope for a good outcome for the relationship.

Recovery has many rewards. One is the ability to look back on a relationship that has grown in ways not thought possible. Being in a relationship with a sex addict has its downsides, to be sure. But when the addict and his or her partner are actively engaged in their own recovery process, and are doing solid work both individually and together, the relationship often possesses a new dimension of richness that could not have occurred were it not for addiction and recovery.

The reason I am committed to providing therapy is because I get to see miracles happen on a daily basis. I continually meet individuals and couples who believe their relationships and their happiness are at an end because of the discovery of addictive sexual behavior. My work with them often proves otherwise.

I am continually amazed at the changes that can take place in relationships through solid recovery work. I regularly hear couples who have been in recovery for several months state that their relationship is better than ever. I have heard this frequently enough that I have come to expect that result when both the sex addict and the partner are committed to doing whatever it takes to restore their relationship.

My desire for you and your partner is that you immerse yourselves in recovery. I urge you to be willing to do the courageous and challenging work that is required. As Francis Bacon once said, "All rising to great places is by a winding stair." May your recovery journey create hope and lead you both to freedom.

APPENDIX A

Intensive Treatment Programs Offered at Hope & Freedom Counseling Services and by Certified Hope & Freedom Practitioners (CHFP)

Note: Certified Hope & Freedom Practitioners (CHFP) are highly skilled sex addiction therapists who have received advanced training and been certified in the Hope & Freedom intensive treatment model to provide the same high-quality Intensives in a variety of convenient locations.

Wallace's Story

Wallace entered recovery after Karen discovered his acting out two years ago. He had done pretty well in recovery and was attending a twelve-step meeting each week and meeting with his sponsor. As far as Karen knew, he had not acted out since entering recovery. She attended her own twelve-step meetings to help her understand how she had missed the signs of her husband's acting out. She learned how to set boundaries as well as develop behaviors that helped her become more emotionally healthy in her recovery.

While their recoveries were going well, their relationship continued to suffer. Karen realized that she was not trusting Wallace and not sure that she had the complete truth about his past acting-out behavior. They applied for admission to the Three-Day Intensive program at Hope & Freedom Counseling Services to rebuild their relationship and ensure they each remained on track with their recovery.

Among the most important and unique forms of therapy we offer at Hope & Freedom Counseling Services are Three-Day Intensives. These brief but highly concentrated periods of treatment that focus on specific aspects of recovery are particularly helpful for individuals or couples first entering recovery. They are an ideal forum in which to deal with the crisis that may have precipitated the recovery process. Intensives are also of great value for anyone who has experienced a slip or relapse or been unable to maintain longer-term recovery.

Three-Day Intensives are not a "Three-Day Cure." There is no such thing. Rather, this is a three-day period for doing intensive recovery work and developing a solid foundation for recovery. Each Intensive is the equivalent of about twenty-four therapy sessions, or approximately six months of weekly therapy. Hope & Freedom Counseling Services offers a variety of Three-Day Intensives that are especially valuable for persons who live in geographical areas where sex addiction therapy is not available.

These are not the treatment choice for every individual or couple where problematic sexual behavior or sex addiction is a factor. If there is significant initial resistance on the part of a couple or an individual, Three-Day Intensives are not indicated. We accept fewer couples than apply for this treatment program, and there are a number of factors that may exclude this as the treatment option of choice.

Persons considering a Three-Day Intensive must be willing to work hard. They must be prepared to do whatever is necessary to stop the destructive behaviors related to sex addiction and be willing to take extraordinary steps to restore their relationship. We ask couples who come to Intensives to be willing to devote total effort to recovery for the three days. That includes not conducting business as usual during the Intensive. We also ask that contacts with home and family be minimized for the duration of the Intensive. For the Intensive process to be successful, it requires couples to be willing to participate in the full three-day experience, including the rigorous assignments that are given each evening. In short, the Intensives we offer work best for highly motivated clients. If a person is not highly motivated, he or she would probably do well to choose another level of treatment.

A prerequisite for participating in an Intensive is for both partners to be stable emotionally. Clients with untreated obsessive-compulsive disorder, bipolar disorder, or severe attention deficit hyperactivity disorder may not be good candidates for Intensives. After these disorders are stabilized with medication and therapy, these persons may be ready for the rigorous Intensive process. Additionally, persons at risk of harming themselves or others are not appropriate for Intensives. (Couples who are not appropriate for Three-Day Intensives may do well in longer intensive outpatient programs or inpatient treatment. Appendix B gives a listing of these treatment providers.)

Couples who are approved for participation in Three-Day Intensives must make a commitment to stay in the relationship after the Intensive. This is crucial, since disclosures typically reveal additional acting-out behaviors or some details about previously known events. This new information often traumatizes (or further traumatizes) the partner. When the pain associated with trauma starts, the typical response is to look to anything to stop the pain, including ending the relationship.

We ask partners to make an unqualified commitment to stay in the relationship for a minimum of twelve months after the Intensive, regardless of what the disclosure reveals. We ask sex addicts to double the commitment and to stay in the relationship a minimum of twenty-four months after the Intensive, regardless of their partner's anger or disappointment. Couples must agree to that in writing in order to participate in the Hope & Freedom Three-Day Intensive program.

People interested in Intensives must first complete an online application and then need to be carefully screened to make sure they are appropriate for an Intensive, and also that there is a reasonable expectation that they will benefit from it. The content of the Intensive is customized to the specific needs of each client or couple. If the client is in a committed relationship, we will only work with him or her as a couple, because successful recovery depends on both partners being involved in the recovery process. (Information and applications about Intensives may be found at www.hopeandfreedom.com.) The following is a partial list of Intensives offered through Hope & Freedom Counseling Services.

RECOVERY FOUNDATIONS INTENSIVE

Recovery Foundations Intensives are designed for men and couples at the beginning of the recovery process, and focus on giving participants a broad understanding of sex addiction and what is involved in recovery. The emphasis is on understanding the origins of addiction and the factors that contribute specifically to sex addiction. These Intensives focus on integrating recovery routines into the couple's relationship as well as reestablishing trust. Relapse prevention is also a significant focus. The Recovery Foundations Intensive culminates with each client drafting a Personal Recovery Plan.

RESTORATION INTENSIVE FOR COUPLES

This Intensive is structured for couples wherein the client has been in recovery a while but has had a slip or a relapse. Attention is given to understanding the cause of the relapse and preventing further relapses. A significant focus of this Intensive is dealing with the issue of trust. The couple is introduced to a process of trust-rebuilding that requires significant commitment from each partner.

SURVIVORS INTENSIVE FOR COUPLES OR FOR INDIVIDUALS

This Intensive is designed for couples wherein one or both partners have experienced significant trauma. The trauma may go back to childhood or be recent, resulting from current sexual acting out. This Intensive focuses on each partner healing around his or her trauma and looking at the impact of the trauma on the relationship. A similar Intensive is offered for individuals.

STEP-DOWN INTENSIVE FOR COUPLES OR FOR INDIVIDUALS

This Intensive is designed as a step-down treatment for couples wherein the sex addict has recently returned from inpatient treatment or from an extended intensive outpatient treatment program. The emphasis is on learning to identify and deal with daily triggers, as well as learning new thought and behavior patterns to replace dysfunctional thoughts and behaviors. Relapse prevention and developing a Personal Recovery Plan round out this Intensive.

SPECIAL TOPIC INTENSIVES

We offer Special Topic Intensives designed to fit specific client needs. These deal with a number of topics related to recovery, including, but not limited to, multiple forms of addiction, couples where the husband and the wife both struggle with addiction, recovery issues involving the family, and religious abuse.

HIGH-PROFILE CLIENT INTENSIVE

Individuals in the public eye face special challenges when entering recovery. If they go into a therapy office, they risk revealing their struggle with some sexual behavior. To address this concern, we take the Intensive to the client. This Intensive is designed for any high-profile person including senior executives, professional athletes, politicians, actors, broadcast personalities, and other celebrities. These are offered at a private location in the United States or Canada. The content is customized to fit the needs of the individual or couple. The location is chosen to allow for an extra buffer of anonymity that is not available for celebrities who enter other treatment centers.

Additional Intensives are offered to meet the special needs of physicians and clergy. These Intensives are highly individualized to deal with the specific issues involved. In cases where an extra level of anonymity is needed, we offer Intensives at locations other than our main site.

AFTERCARE INTENSIVES

A rigorous aftercare program is an important ingredient in any recovery treatment program. After the initial three days of work, we encourage couples to come back for periodic one-day Aftercare Intensives. These are mini-versions of a Three-Day Intensive. During the Aftercare Intensives, couples have a combination of individual and couples therapy. The Aftercare Intensives are used to check up on recovery progress, and for the couple to learn additional tools of recovery and work on communication issues they may be facing. A follow-up polygraph exam is offered and strongly suggested to verify that acting out has not recurred.

The first of these one-day follow-ups is scheduled three months after the Three-Day Intensive. They are then scheduled every six months for an additional eighteen to thirty-six months, depending on the couple's need. Thereafter we encourage couples to schedule an Aftercare Intensive annually as a checkup on the relationship and to monitor progress in recovery.

APPENDIX B
RESOURCE GUIDE

Twelve-Step Programs Dedicated to Helping Sex Addicts

- Sex and Love Addicts Anonymous (SLAA), 210-828-7900, www.slaafws.org
- Sex Addicts Anonymous (SAA), 713-869-4902 or 800-477-8191, www.sexaa.org
- Sexual Compulsives Anonymous (SCA), 800-977-4325, www.sca-recovery.org
- Sexaholics Anonymous (SA), 866-424-8777, www.sa.org
- Sexual Recovery Anonymous (SRA), NY: 646-450-9690 or CA: 323-850-8565, www.sexualrecovery.org

Twelve-Step Programs Dedicated to Helping the Spouses and Partners of Sex Addicts

- Infidelity Survivors Anonymous (ISA), www.isurvivors.org
- S-Anon, 615-833-3152, www.sanon.org
- Co-Dependents of Sex Addicts (COSA), 866-899-2672, www.cosa-recovery.org

Twelve-Step Programs Dedicated to Helping Couples

- Recovering Couples Anonymous (RCA), 877-663-2317, www.recovering-couples.org

Intensive Outpatient Sex Addiction Treatment Programs

Center for Healthy Sex

• Intensive programs for men, women, and couples with the goal of moving clients into healthy sexuality.

9911 W. Pico Blvd., Suite 700
Los Angeles, CA 90035
www.thecenterforhealthysex.com
310-843-9902

Hope & Freedom Counseling Services

• Individualized Three-Day Intensives for couples and for men.

• Special programs available for physicians and clergy.

• Celebrity intensives at a resort setting in the Canadian Rockies or at other confidential locations in North America.

3730 Kirby Dr., Suite 1130
Houston, TX 77098
www.hopeandfreedom.com
713-630-0111

Certified Hope & Freedom Practitioners (CHFP)

• These sex addiction therapists are certified in the Hope & Freedom intensive treatment model and offer Intensives in a variety of locations. A listing of these clinicians can be found at:

www.hopeandfreedom.com and
www.hopeandfreedom.net

Psychological Counseling Services (PCS)

• One- to four-week intensive outpatient programs for men, women, and couples, with a heavy focus on individual therapy.

7530 E. Angus Dr.
Scottsdale, AZ 85251
www.pcsearle.com
480-947-5739

Sexual Recovery Institute (SRI)

• Two-week intensive outpatient programs for men, women, and spouses.

914 S. Robertson Blvd., Suite 200
Los Angeles, CA 90035
www.sexualrecovery.com
866-585-9174

Inpatient Sex Addiction Treatment Centers

Del Amo Hospital

23700 Camino del Sol
Torrance, CA 90505
www.delamohospital.com
800-824-4936

Gentle Path at Pine Grove

2255 Broadway Dr.
Hattiesburg, MS 39402
www.pinegrovetreatment.com
888-574-4673

Keystone Center

2000 Providence Ave.
Chester, PA 19013
www.keystonecenterecu.net
800-733-6840

Life Healing Center

25 Vista Point Rd.
Santa Fe, NM 87506
www.life-healing.com
866-806-7214

The Meadows

1655 N. Tegner St.
Wickenburg, AZ 85390
www.themeadows.org
800-632-3697

Sante Center for Healing

914 Country Club Rd.
Argyle, TX 76226
www.santecenter.com
800-258-4250

Sierra Tucson, Inc.

39580 S. Lago del Oro Pkwy
Tucson, AZ 85739
www.sierratucson.com
800-842-4487

Websites for Therapists Who Specialize in Sex Addiction

• The International Institute for Trauma and Addiction Professionals: www.iitap.com

• The Society for the Advancement of Sexual Health: www.sash.net

Christian-Based Workshops

Bethesda Workshops

• Workshops for men, women, and couples.

3710 Franklin Pike
Nashville, TN 37204
www.bethesdaworkshops.org
866-464-4325

Be Broken Ministries
• Workshops for men, women, and couples.

19115 FM 2252, Ste. 8
Garden Ridge, TX 78266
www.bebroken.com
800-497-8748

Faithful & True Ministries
• Three-day workshops for men, women, and couples.

15798 Venture Ln.
Eden Prairie, MN 55344
www.faithfulandtrue.com
952-746-3880

Journey of Hope Men's Retreats
• Hope & Freedom offers heavily subsidized retreats each year as a gift to the recovery community.

www.hopeandfreedom.com

Sex Addiction Recovery-Related Websites

www.journeytohealingandjoy.com
Telephone support groups for partners of sex addicts. They have recently expanded to offer telephone support groups for sex addicts as well. They take a Christian approach to recovery. This site offers telephone-based support groups for partners of sex addicts that focus on trauma resolution.

www.celebritysexaddict.com
Intensive outpatient programs for persons who cannot visit a therapist without becoming the subject of media scrutiny.

www.gottostopit.com
A YouTube channel with many videos related to sex addiction and recovery.

www.guardyoureyes.com
For Jews who struggle with problematic sexual behavior.

www.hopeandfreedom.com
Resources for persons wanting to learn about sex addiction.

www.hopeandfreedom.net
Training offered for therapists with significant experience in treating sex addiction who want to be trained in the Hope & Freedom treatment model to become Certified Hope & Freedom Practitioners (CHFP).

www.hopeandfreedomu.com
Online sex addiction recovery education that includes streaming video courses.

www.internetbehavior.com
Provides cybersex addiction research and resources. This site also includes a screening exam for persons who think they may be addicted to cybersex behavior.

www.physiciansincrisis.com
Intensive outpatient therapy for physicians who struggle with sex addiction.

www.ldshopeandrecovery.com
Resources for persons who are members of the Church of Jesus Christ of Latter Day Saints.

www.recoveryapp.com
Recovery-related applications for smartphones, iPads, and other platforms.

www.recoveryonthego.com
Brief audiobooks and MP3 downloads for getting started in recovery.

www.saatalk.org
Gives a list of SAA meetings that take place by electronic means.

www.sexhelp.com
This site also offers a screening exam for anyone who wonders if he or she might be a sex addict.

www.woundedclergy.com
Brief intensive programs for clergy struggling with sex addiction. (Please be advised that this website is actually a page on the Hope & Freedom site.)

Twelve-Step Programs for Other Compulsive Behaviors and Forms of Addiction

Alcoholics Anonymous
www.aa.org

Cocaine Anonymous
www.ca.org

Crystal Meth Anonymous
www.crystalmeth.org

Debtors Anonymous
www.debtorsanonymous.org

Food Addicts Anonymous
www.foodaddictsanonymous.org

Gamblers Anonymous
www.gamblersanonymous.org

Marijuana Anonymous
www.marijuana-anonymous.org

Narcotics Anonymous
www.na.org

Nicotine Anonymous
www.nicotine-anonymous.org

Overeaters Anonymous
www.oa.org

Spenders Anonymous
www.spenders.org

Shopaholics Anonymous
www.shopaholicsanonymous.org

Workaholics Anonymous
www.workaholics-anonymous.org

Additional Web-Based Resources

iRecovery Addiction Recovery Tracker

This iPhone application is designed to keep track of recovery activities and plot the user's progress. The tracking process is also designed to be an encouragement to think about recovery daily.

- Assigns recovery points to typical recovery activities.

- Charts those activities and compares progress from week to week.

- Users can add their activities and assign a point value for each.

- Will send weekly accountability emails to Circle of Five and therapist/counselor showing progress for the week.

- "Call Sponsor" button visible on every screen for immediate contact with sponsor.

- Preloaded affirmations with counter.

- Users can also add their own affirmations.

- User-defined Red Light, Yellow Light, and Green Light behaviors.

- Contacts button takes users to list of their Circle of Five contacts.

- Recovery points can be customized to meet individual recovery plans as directed by counselor or therapist.

- www.recoveryapp.com

Recovery on the Go

Audio messages, each approximately twenty minutes in length, dealing with the following areas:

1. Am I a Sex Addict?
2. Lost in Cyber Space
3. Intensive Preparation for Her
4. Intensive Preparation for Him
5. Getting Started in Recovery I
6. Getting Started in Recovery II
7. Disclosure
8. Accountability in Recovery

These audio messages are particularly beneficial when the sex addict or partner could benefit from a therapist giving reinforcement for the path he or she is taking to freedom from addiction.

THE TWELVE STEPS OF SEX ADDICTS ANONYMOUS[41]

1. We admitted we were powerless over addictive sexual behavior—that our lives had become unmanageable.

2. Came to believe that a Power greater than ourselves could restore us to sanity.

3. Made a decision to turn our will and our lives over to the care of God as we understood God.

4. Made a searching and fearless moral inventory of ourselves.

5. Admitted to God, to ourselves, and to another human being the exact nature of our wrongs.

6. Were entirely ready to have God remove all these defects of character.

7. Humbly asked God to remove our shortcomings.

8. Made a list of all persons we had harmed and became willing to make amends to them all.

9. Made direct amends to such people wherever possible, except when to do so would injure them or others.

10. Continued to take personal inventory and when we were wrong promptly admitted it.

11. Sought through prayer and meditation to improve our conscious contact with God as we understood God, praying only for knowledge of God's will for us and the power to carry that out.

12. Having had a spiritual awakening as the result of these steps, we tried to carry this message to other sex addicts and to practice these principles in our lives.

BIBLIOGRAPHY AND SUGGESTED READING

Alcoholics Anonymous, Fourth Edition. (2002). New York: Alcoholics Anonymous World Services, Inc.

American Heritage Dictionary, Third Edition. (1992). Boston: Houghton Mifflin.

Black, C. (2009). *Deceived: Facing Sexual Betrayal, Lies, and Secrets.* Center City, MN: Hazelden.

Black, C., and Tripodi, C. (2012). *Intimate Treason: Healing the Trauma for Partners Confronting Sex Addiction.* Las Vegas: Central Recovery Press.

Canning, M. (2008). *Lust, Anger, Love: Understanding Sexual Addiction and the Road to Healthy Intimacy.* Naperville, IL: Sourcebooks.

Carnes, P. (2001). *Out of the Shadows: Starting Sexual and Relationship Recovery.* Center City, MN: Hazelden.

Cooper, A. (2000). *Cybersex: The Dark Side of the Force.* London: Taylor Frances.

Diagnostic and Statistical Manual of Mental Disorders, Fourth Edition. (1994). Text Revision. Washington, DC: American Psychiatric Association.

DSM-5 Development. (2010). http://www.dsm5.org/ProposedRevisions/ Pages/proposedrevision.aspx?rid=415 (Accessed February 10, 2010). Washington, DC: American Psychiatric Association.

Earle, R., and Earle, M. (1995). *Sex Addiction: Case Studies and Management*. New York: Brunner/Mazel.

Edwards, W., Delmonico, D., and Griffin, E. (2011). *Cybersex Unplugged: Finding Sexual Health in an Electronic World*. Seattle, WA: CreateSpace Independent Publishing.

Ferree, M. (2002). *No Stones: Women Redeemed from Sexual Shame*. Maitland, FL: Xulon Press.

Ferree, M. ed. (2012). *Making Advances: A Comprehensive Guide for Treating Female Sex and Love Addicts*. Royston, GA: Society for the Advancement of Sexual Health.

Laaser, D. (2008). *Shattered Vows: Hope and Healing for Women Who Have Been Sexually Betrayed*. Grand Rapids, MI: Zondervan.

Laaser, M. (2004). *Healing the Wounds of Sexual Addiction*. Grand Rapids, MI: Zondervan.

Magness, M. (2012). *I Can Stop: The 30 Day Solution to Sex Addiction*. DVD Series. H&F Media.

Magness, M. (2013). *I Must Heal: Healing from Your Partner's Sex Addiction*. DVD Series. H&F Media.

McDaniel, K. (2009). *Ready to Heal: Breaking Free of Addictive Relationships, Third Edition*. Carefree, AZ: Gentle Path Press.

Mellody, P. (1989). *Facing Codependence: What It Is, Where It Comes From, How It Sabotages Our Lives*. New York: HarperCollins.

Schneider, J., and Corley, D. (2012). *Disclosing Secrets: A Sex Addict's Guide for When, to Whom, and How Much to Reveal*. Seattle, WA: CreateSpace Independent Publishing.

Schneider, J., and Corley, D. (2012). *Surviving Disclosure: A Partner's Guide for Healing the Betrayal of Intimate Trust*. Seattle, WA: CreateSpace Independent Publishing.

Schneider, J. (2005). *Back from Betrayal: Recovering from His Affairs*. Tucson, AZ: Recovery Resources Press.

Sex Addicts Anonymous, Second Edition. (2008). Houston, TX: Sex Addicts Anonymous.

Steffens, B., and Means, M. (2009). *Your Sexually Addicted Spouse: How Partners Can Cope and Heal.* Far Hills, NJ: New Horizon Press.

ENDNOTES

1   http://Internet-filter-review-toptenreviews.com/Internet-pornography-statistics.html (Accessed March 15, 2012).

2   G. Burke, "North America – United States – Christianity – Catholic" (March 18, 2009), from *World Wide Religious News:* www.uurn.org (Accessed March 4, 2012).

3   R. Taylor, "Sex-Trade Workers Trafficked Around the World," from suite101.com: http://human-rights-violations.suite101.com (Accessed December 4, 2011).

4   Centers for Disease Control and Prevention, "Annual CDC Report Finds High Burden of Sexually Transmitted Diseases, Especially Among Women and Racial Minorities" (January, 2009). www.cdc.gov (Accessed December 4, 2011).

5   www.sash.net (Accessed March 2, 2012).

6   American Psychiatric Association, *Diagnostic and Statistical Manual of Mental Disorders* (Fourth Edition, Text Revision). Washington, DC: American Psychiatric Association, 2000.

7   Society for the Advancement of Sexual Health, "Sexual Addiction," www.sash.net (Accessed March 15, 2012).

8   http://www.familysafemedia.com/pornography_statistics.html (Accessed February 23, 2012).

9   Telephone survey was conducted October 7–14, 2010. The calling list was randomly drawn from a list of all Protestant churches. Up to six calls were made to reach a sampled phone number. Interviews were conducted with the senior pastor, minister, or priest of the church called. Responses were weighted to reflect the geographic distribution of Protestant churches. The sample provides 95 percent confidence that the sampling error does not exceed plus or minus 3.2 percent. http://www.lifeway.com/LifeWay-Research/c/N-1z13wgl (Accessed April 22, 2012).

10 A. Cooper, *Cybersex: The Dark Side of the Force*. Philadelphia, PA: Brunner-Routledge.

11 The National Campaign to Prevent Teen and Unplanned Pregnancy, "Sex and Tech: Results from a Survey of Teens and Young Adults" (January 15, 2009), www.thenationalcampaign.org (Accessed March 12, 2011).

12 www.celebritysexaddict.com gives information about a treatment program that provides for complete privacy and anonymity for high-profile persons.

13 A much more detailed look at the behaviors necessary for recovery are found in M. Magness, *Thirty Days to Hope & Freedom from Sexual Addiction: The Essential Guide to Beginning Recovery and Preventing Relapse*. Carefree, AZ: Gentle Path Press, 2011.

14 American Psychiatric Association, *Diagnostic and Statistical Manual of Mental Disorders*.

15 A more lengthy discussion of the problems caused by denial and resistance is found in M. Magness, *Thirty Days to Hope & Freedom from Sexual Addiction*.

16 Romans 7: 18–19, NLT.

17 *American Heritage Dictionary*, Third Edition, 1992.

18 *Alcoholics Anonymous*, Fourth Edition. Alcoholics Anonymous World Services, Inc., 2002, p. 58.

[19] J. Schneider, D. Corley, and R. Irons, "Surviving Disclosure of Infidelity: Results of an International Survey of 164 Recovering Sex Addicts and Their Partners," *Sexual Addiction & Compulsivity* (1998): pp. 189–217.

[20] Most disclosures at Hope & Freedom Counseling Services are currently done as part of a Three-Day Intensive program. You can read more about Intensives in Appendix A. The process in this chapter is a typical process that is used when a disclosure is conducted utilizing individual therapy each week over a period of several months.

[21] P. Mellody, *Facing Codependence: What It Is, Where It Comes From, How It Sabotages Our Lives.* San Francisco: HarperCollins, 1989.

[22] J. Schneider, D. Corley, and R. Irons, "Surviving Disclosure of Infidelity," pp. 189–217.

[23] The complete results of this study are found in M. Magness, *Thirty Days to Hope & Freedom from Sexual Addiction.*

[24] Stephen Cabler's website is www.cablerpolygraphllc.com.

[25] B. Steffens and M. Means, *Your Sexually Addicted Spouse: How Partners Can Cope and Heal.* Far Hills, NJ: New Horizon Press, 2009.

[26] J. Schneider, D. Corley, and R. Irons, "Surviving Disclosure of Infidelity," pp. 189–217.

[27] K. Coop-Gordon, D. Baucom, and D. Snyder, "An Integrative Intervention for Promoting Recovery from Extra Marital Affairs," *Journal of Marital and Family Therapy* (2004): p. 213.

[28] B. Steffens and R. Rennie, "The Traumatic Nature of Disclosure for Wives of Sexual Addicts," *Sexual Addiction and Compulsivity* (2006): pp. 247–267.

[29] EMDR Institute, Inc., "Eye Movement Desensitization and Reprocessing," www.emdr.com (Accessed August 4, 2011).

[30] B. Steffens and M. Means, *Your Sexually Addicted Spouse.*

31 The concept of adopting recovery as a lifestyle is explored fully in M. Magness, *Thirty Days to Hope & Freedom for Sexual Addicts*.

32 A listing of CSATs and those working toward certification can be found at www.iitap.com.

33 This system is explained in depth in M. Magness, *Thirty Days to Hope & Freedom from Sexual Addiction*.

34 www.womanwithin.org.

35 One of the most effective ways of describing the activities of recovery is to utilize the Recovery Points System detailed in M. Magness, *Thirty Days to Hope & Freedom from Sexual Addiction*. There is also a smartphone app called iRecovery that utilizes the Recovery Points System.

36 *Sex Addicts Anonymous*, 2005, p. 68.

37 M. Magness, *Thirty Days to Hope & Freedom from Sexual Addiction* has two chapters that are devoted to tools for dealing with threats to sexual sobriety.

38 The Recovery Points System is discussed at length in M. Magness, *Thirty Days to Hope & Freedom from Sexual Addiction*. Additional Recovery Points Worksheets can be downloaded at www.thirtydaysthebook.com.

39 *Alcoholics Anonymous, Fourth Edition*, Alcoholics Anonymous World Services, Inc., 2002, pp. 58–59.

40 Ibid., pp. 83–84.

41 Copyright by the International Service Organization of Sex Addicts Anonymous.